SEXUAL DIMORPHISM

Edited by **Hiroshi Moriyama**

Sexual Dimorphism
http://dx.doi.org/10.5772/2960
Edited by Hiroshi Moriyama

Contributors

Chelsea M. Berns, Angel Alonso Romero-López, Miguel Angel Morón, Hugo A. Benítez, Hirokazu Ozawa, Katsumasa Muneoka, Makiko Kuwagata, Freddy Moreno-Gómez, Hiroshi Moriyama

Published by InTech
Janeza Trdine 9, 51000 Rijeka, Croatia

Notice

Publishing Process Manager Oliver Kurelic
Technical Editor InTech Prepress, Novi Sad
Cover InTech Design team

Additional hard copies can be obtained from orders@intechopen.com

Sexual Dimorphism, Edited by Hiroshi Moriyama
p. cm.
ISBN 978-953-51-1075-0

For EU product safety concerns:
IN TECH d.o.o., Prolaz Marije Krucifikse Kozulić 3, 51000 Rijeka, Croatia,
info@intechopen.com or visit our website at intechopen.com.

Meet the editor

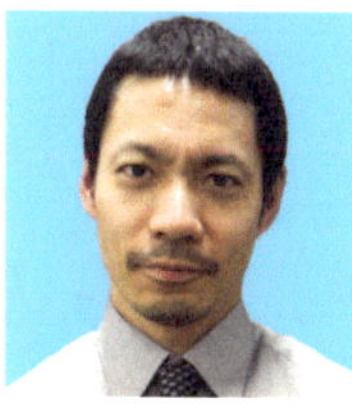

Dr. Moriyama is an Associate Professor, Section of Gross Anatomy, Department of Anatomy, Showa University School of Medicine, Tokyo Japan. He is also a Visiting Lecturer, Tokyo Medical University, Nippon Dental University, and Kanagawa Dental College. He received his DDS degree from Matsumoto Dental University and his PhD degree from Showa University School of Medicine. He was part of the Attending Staff in Anesthesiology from 1986 to 1990. He has been studying clinical anatomy since 1991. He has served on the Editorial Boards of The Scientific World Journal, International Journal of Medical Imaging, Clinical Medicine Research and Science Journal of Clinical Medicine. His research interests include morphometry of peripheral nerves and muscles, and the development, aging process, sex difference, and asymmetry of human organs.

Contents

Preface

The first scientist to raise scientific questions about sex differences was Charles Robert Darwin, as part of his research into differences among members of the same species. Since Darwin's research, many scientists have studied sex differences and concluded that there are two different states for females and males. One is the sex difference, which is biological and congenital, based on genes and completed by hormones. The other difference is gender, which is social, cultural, acquired, not based on genes, but rather shaped by environmental factors. Scientists have argued whether the differences between females and males are innate or occur after birth, when differences are influenced by the environment, that is to say - "Nature or Nurture". For example, Sigmund Freud made the famous remark "Anatomy is destiny", whereas Simone de Beauvoir claimed that "One is not born a woman, but becomes one." I do not believe that females and males are shaped solely by nature or nurture; rather, I believe that they are formed out of the interaction between nature and nurture. Therefore, this book offers new ideas not only to life scientists and biologists, but also to social and cultural scientists.

It has become clear in recent years that sex differences and similarities in biology have influenced physiological and pathological functions. However, there have been few reports on intentional studies of sex differences, and many reports have been published as by-products of other kinds of research. Sex difference specialists in their own respective fields contributed to this book. They have chosen not only humans as the subjects of their studies, but other mammals, birds, amphibians, insects, and extended the scope to ostracoda in the Paleozoic era. Moreover, they have used original methods in individual studies. My own contribution offers somewhat different data on sex differences to readers.

Nowadays, studies in life science are not complete without factoring in sex differences. Researchers have been exploring new medical treatments under the assumption that physical characteristics in females are different from those in males. I hope that this book will be able to contribute to the advancement of life science and the progress of gender-specific medicine.

I offer my thanks to the production team at InTech, under the leadership of Oliver Kurelic and Natalia Reinic, for their guidance, professionalism and unfailing support.

In what has truly been a team effort, it is difficult to single out individuals for special mention.

I am also grateful to Ikuko Moriyama, librarian and my long-suffering wife, for assistance in preparing the manuscript, and her patience and tolerance throughout the last two years.

Hiroshi Moriyama
Showa University
School of Medicine
Japan

Chapter 1

The Evolution of Sexual Dimorphism: Understanding Mechanisms of Sexual Shape Differences

Chelsea M. Berns

Additional information is available at the end of the chapter

http://dx.doi.org/10.5772/55154

1. Introduction

Understanding the origin of biodiversity has been a major focus in evolutionary and ecological biology for well over a century and several patterns and mechanisms have been proposed to explain this diversity. Particularly intriguing is the pattern of sexual dimorphism, in which males and females of the same species differ in some trait. Sexual dimorphism (SD) is a pattern that is seen throughout the animal kingdom and is exhibited in a myriad of ways. For example, differences between the sexes in coloration are common in many organisms [1] ranging from poeciliid fishes [2] to dragon flies [3] to eclectus parrots (see Figure 1).

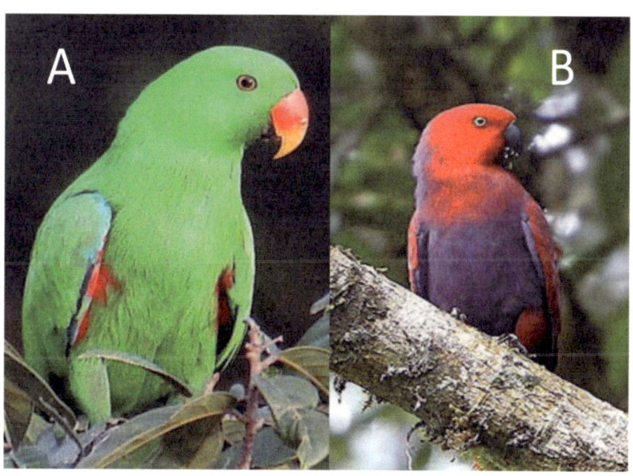

Figure 1. A) Male Eclectus (© Stijn De Win/Birding2asia)
B) Female Eclectus (© James Eaton/Birdtour Asia)

Sexual dimorphism is also exhibited in ornamentation, such as the horns of dung beetles [4], the antlers of cervids [5], and the tail of peacocks [6]. Many species also exhibit sexual differences in foraging behavior such as the Russian agamid lizard [7], and parental behavior and territoriality can be dimorphic in species such as hummingbirds [8, 9]. Another common pattern is that of sexual size dimorphism, such as is observed in snakes [10] and monk seals [11].

There are many mechanisms that drive the evolution of SD, the most accepted mechanism being sexual selection [12-14], which enhances fitness of each sex exclusively in relation to reproduction [15, 16]. This states that SD evolves in a direction such that each sex (especially males, see 17) maximizes reproductive success in two ways: by becoming more attractive to the other sex (inter-sexual dimorphism) or by enhancing the ability to defeat same-sex rivals (intra-sexual dimorphism), in both cases such that each sex increases the chances to mate and pass genes on to the next generation. Many researchers have argued that competition for mates is at the very heart of sexual selection because these rivalries greatly influence mating and fertilization success. Indeed, competition for mates has been shown to be the major factor impacting SD in several taxa [18]. However the complexity of SD cannot be explained by a single mechanism.

Mate choice is an important proximate mechanism of sexual selection. Often the sex with the higher reproductive investment is the 'choosy' sex. Patterns then emerge, such as those consistent with the 'sexy son' hypothesis [19], where females prefer mates with phenotypes signifying fitness. The females prefer males that are phenotypically 'sexy' to ensure that the genes of their offspring will produce males that will have the most breeding success, propagating her genes successfully [16, 20]. Taken further, sometimes females prefer males that exhibit very extreme phenotypes within a population. Over evolutionary time these traits become increasingly exaggerated despite the potential fitness costs to the males themselves, termed Fisherian runaway sexual selection [19]. Examples include the tails of male peacocks, plumage in birds of paradise and male insect genitalia [14, 21, 22].

Alternatively, ecological mechanisms, such as competition for resources, may exert distinct selective forces on the sexes resulting in the evolution of SD [23]. Here, intraspecific competition in species-poor communities may allow divergent selection between the sexes (rather than between species), resulting in sexual niche segregatation [12, 24-26]. In this case morphological traits often change to minimize this intersexual competition. Other ecological hypotheses have been proposed to explain patterns of SD, such as the influence of sex-specific divergence in response to environmental gradients (i.e., intersexual niche packing: sensu 27]. For example, both sexes of fruit flies *Drosophila subobscura* increase in body size with latitude, however in South America these size increases are less steep and weaker in males as compared to females [28]. Another study found weaker latitudinal clines in males as compared to females in houseflies *Musca domestica* [29], and yet another study found geographical variation in climate that corresponded to a change in the magnitude of sexual size dimorphism between males and females [30]. Hypotheses continue to be proposed and the explanations for the evolution of SD may not be mutually exclusive but instead, may operate in a synergistic or antagonist fashion to shape these patterns.

2. Processes and patterns of sexual size dimorphism

Sexual size dimorphism is a frequent phenomenon where the size of males and females of the same species differ (see Figure 2), driven by one or more of the mechanisms mentioned above. When these processes occur in closely related species, distinct patterns of among-species size dimorphism can result, one of which is termed 'Rensch's Rule' [31]. Rensch's rule is a pattern wherein the degree of sexual size dimorphism increases with body size in species where males are the larger sex, and conversely decreases in those species where females are the larger sex (see Figure 3).

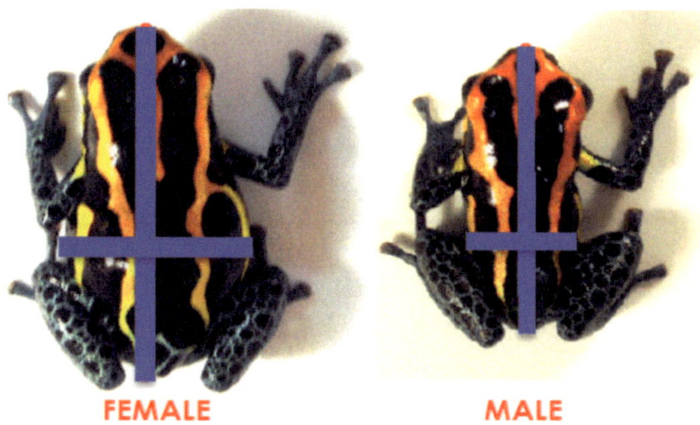

Photograph by: http://www.joshsfrogs.com/catalog/blog/category/poison-dart-frog-care

Figure 2. Sexual size dimorphism in poison dart frog.

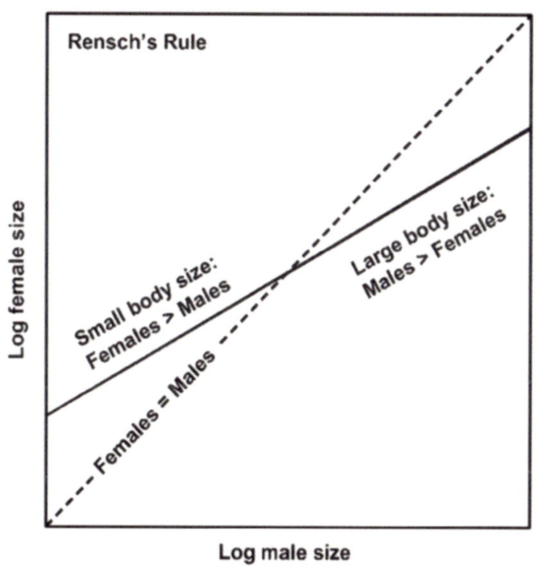

Figure 3. Rensch's Rule, where in species above the broken line (broken line denoting where female and male sizes are equal) females are larger than males and below, males are larger than females. From R. Colwell, Am. Nat., 2000.

Several hypotheses have been proposed to explain Rensch's rule. One proposes that the combination of genetic correlations between male and female size with directional sexual selection for larger male size will cause the evolution of larger males relative to female body size [13, 32, 33]. Another argues that sexual size dimorphism evolves through intraspecific competition between the sexes when foraging is related to size [15, 26]. Finally, many researchers have hypothesized that this pattern is due to female fecundity, where the larger female will have bigger eggs and a greater capacity to reproduce successfully [15, 34, 35]. Examples of Rensch's rule and support for all three hypotheses abound in nature in organisms as diverse as hummingbirds [36], hummingbird flower mites [36], water striders [32], turtles [37], salmon [38] and shorebirds [39].

Another such pattern is that of 'adaptive canalization', where the larger sex has less plasticity compared to the smaller sex. This is due to directional selection for a large body size and individuals with sub-optimal body sizes will have lower fitness [40, 41]. Alternatively, there may be condition-dependence, where the larger sex is under stronger directional selection for a large size and will be more affected by different environmental factors as compared to the smaller sex. This indicates that sexual size dimorphism should change with changing environments. These hypotheses and studies have led to much understanding of the patterns and processes underlying sexual size dimorphism.

3. Sexual shape dimorphism

In addition to sexual size dimorphism, males and females often differ widely in shape [42, 43]. Curiously, although shape can contribute meaningfully to various functions such as feeding, mating, parental care and other life history characteristics, patterns of sexual shape dimorphism have historically received considerably less attention than sexual size differences [12, 44, 45, 46]. Examining the size and shape of traits together provides a much more complete quantification of sexual dimorphism, as the two components are necessarily related to one another. As such, shape analysis allows a deeper understanding of mechanisms underlying SD, because different parts of the body can serve multiple functions and be under distinct selective regimes.

Shape is defined as the specific form of a distinct object that is invariant to changes in position, rotation and scale [46, 47], and many methods have been proposed to study shape. For instance, sets of linear distances may be measured on each individual (e.g., length, width and height) to represent shape (Figure 4A), as well as angles (Figure 4B) and ratios of these measurements.

Sets of linear distances do not always accurately capture shape because of shortcomings that limit their general utility. For instance, it is possible that for some objects the same set of distance measurements may be obtained from two different shapes, because the location of the measurements is not recorded in the distance measures themselves. For example, if the maximum length and width were taken on an oval and teardrop, the linear values might be the same even though the shapes are clearly different (see Figure 5). Additionally, it is not possible to generate graphical representations of shape using these measurements alone because the geometric distances among variables is not preserved and aspects of shape are lost [48]. As a result of these shortcomings, other analytical approaches for quantifying shape have been developed.

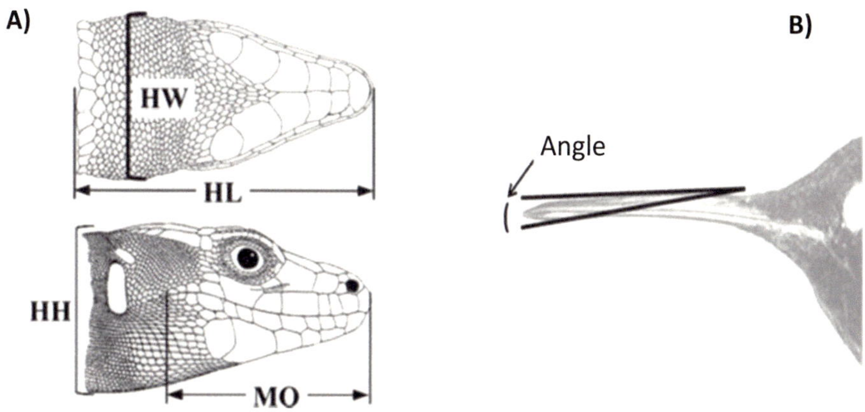

Figure 4. A) Sets of linear distances: Head length (HL), head width (HW), head height (HH), and mouth opening (MO) and B) Measurement of angle. A): adapted from Kaliontzopoulou et al. 2012. B): adapted from Berns and Adams, 2010

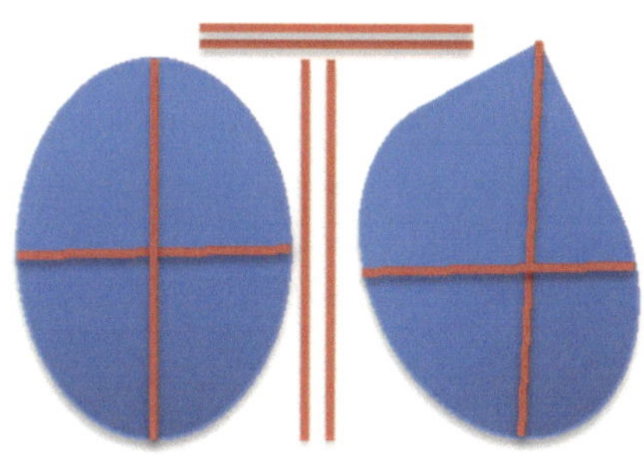

Figure 5. Maximum height and width taken on two different shapes results in the same linear measurement on both

A major advance in the study of shape is landmark-based geometric morphometric methods, which do not have these difficulties. These methods quantify the shape of anatomical objects using the Cartesian coordinates of biologically homologous landmarks whose location is identified on each specimen (Figure 6). These landmarks can be digitized in either two- or three-dimensions, and provide a means of shape quantification that enables graphical representations of shape (see below).

Geometric morphometric analyses of shape are accomplished in several sequential steps. First, the landmark coordinates are digitized from each specimen. Next, differences in specimen position, orientation and size are eliminated through a generalized Procrustes analysis. This procedure translates all specimens to the origin, scales them to unit centroid size, and optimally rotates them to minimize the total sums-of-squares deviations of the landmark coordinates from all specimens to the average configuration. The resulting aligned Procrustes shape coordinates describe the location of each specimen in a curved space related to Kendall's shape space [49, 50]. These are then projected orthogonally onto a linear tangent space yielding Kendall's tangent space coordinates [47, 51, 52], which can then be treated as a set of shape variables for further analyses of shape variation and covariation with other variables [e.g., 53, 54, 55].

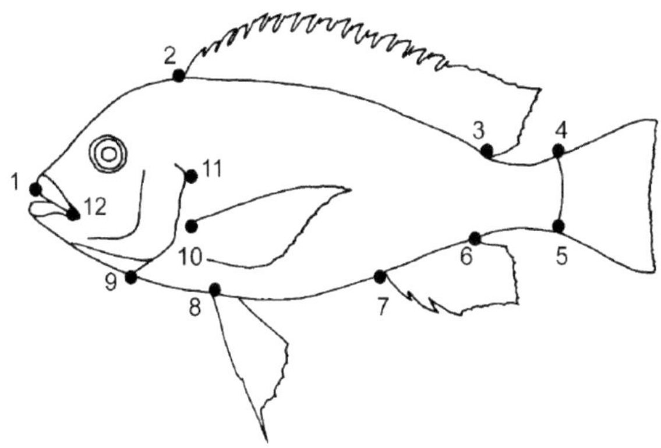

Figure 6. Example of biologically homologous landmarks From Kassam *et al.* 2003

In terms of sexual shape dimorphism, dimorphism, sets of both linear measurements and geometric morphometric methods have been utilized to identify patterns of shape dimorphism in numerous taxa, including fish [56], turtles [57], birds [58-61] and lizards [62, 63]. In addition to quantifying sexual shape dimorphism, identifying the potential mechanisms that generate these patterns is a current focus of many evolutionary biologists. For instance, one central hypothesis for the evolution of sexual shape dimorphism is that males and females diverge phenotypically due to intersexual competition for similar resources. Here, functional morphological traits diverge between the sexes such that the sexes partition resources. Under this scenario, SD is more strongly influenced by natural selection than sexual selection. For example, in the cottonmouth *Agikistrodon piscivorous*, sex-specific prey consumption as a function of prey size is directly correlated with differences in head morphology between males and females [64]. Thus natural selection, and not sexual selection, maintains both foraging and morphological differences between the sexes in this species.

By contrast, sexual shape dimorphism can be the result of sexual selection. For example, in the tuatara *Sphenodon punctatus*, Herrel *et al.* [65] tested the hypothesis that sexual shape dimorphism is due to niche differentiation between the sexes, rather than driven by the territoriality of males. Head shape is much larger in males as compared to females and this may be functionally tied to the larger prey of males. The authors suggested that sexual selection for male-male combat may play a role, but that bite force differences between males and females may be impacting the maintenance of these sexual differences. Interestingly, it was found that males do have a greater bite force relative to females, but that these differences and their maintenance are the result of sexual selection, as bite force is correlated with good male condition but not with female condition [66].

Another study also rejects the hypothesis that differential niches maintain sexual shape dimorphism. Feeding, territory, and mate acquisition have been proposed as functions for the bill of the Cory shearwater *Calonectris diomedea* [61]. The bill morphology is such that sexual differences are related not to feeding ecology, but to sexual selection and antagonistic interactions. On the other hand, the Purple-throated Carib *Eulampis jugularis* hummingbird exhibits the clear link between function and the different food preference of males and females, suggesting that the longer and more curved bill of the female as compared to the male is due to the division of resources [67-69]. In other species of hummingbirds that exhibit sexual size and shape dimorphism in their bills however, it is unclear whether interspecific competition and niche differentiation, sexual selection, or some other force drives this sex-specific morphology [58, 60].

One study investigated the relative contributions of intersexual resource partitioning and sexual selection in the amagid lizard *Japalura swinhonis* [63]. Here, sexual shape dimorphism was not correlated with diet, however limb size and shape were associated with perch habitats. These findings are inconsistent with the hypothesis of intraspecific competition for resources, but provide evidence for the 'fecundity advantage' hypothesis. Under this hypothesis, a large mother can produce more offspring than a small mother, and can give her offspring better conditions through directional selection [14]. For instance, an increase in abdominal volume can arise with an increase in overall body size, seen in some mammals and amphibians [70, 71], or in the abdomen's relative proportion to overall body size, like that of some reptiles [72]. Olsson *et al.* [73] examined SD in the heads and trunk length of an Australian lizard *Niveoscincus microlepidotus* to address the hypothesis that head morphology dimorphism had evolved via sexual selection for male-male combat and that trunk length evolved due to fecundity selection. Results did not uphold one part of this prediction however, as sex divergence in head morphology was genetic and not specifically due to sexual selection. Evidence was presented in favor of the prediction that difference in trunk length is driven by fecundity advantage, and that sexual selection favored males with smaller trunk size. Studies such as these suggest that sexually dimorphic shape traits may be driven by the combination of natural selection for fecundity advantage and by sexual selection.

Evidence supporting fecundity advantage is weak or not existent in many systems however. For instance, investigators examining the tortoise *Testudo horsfieldii* hypothesized that the wider shells of the females provided more room for eggs, but were unable to provide conclusive evidence for fecundity advantage. Instead, the patterns of sexual shape dimorphism seemed to be due primarily to locomotive constraints of mate seeking and male-male combat [74]. In two species of crested newt *Triturus cristatus* and *T. vulgaris,* results somewhat support fecundity advantage, however researchers suggest there are more underlying processes driving the evolution of sexual shape dimorphism than simply fecundity selection [75]. Evidence presented by Willemsen and Haile [76] outright reject the fecundity advantage hypothesis. Three tortoise species *Testudo graeca, T. hermanni,* and *T. marginata* have differing courtship behaviors and display differing magnitudes of sexual shape dimorphism dependent on their specific courtship display. In contrast to previous studies, the authors suggest that these results indicate that sexual shape dimorphism is driven not by fecundity advantage and natural selection, but rather by sexual selection. From the inconcordant results of studies such as these, it remains unknown whether patterns of the evolution of sexual shape dimorphism are primarily driven by natural selection for fecundity advantage or by some other mechanism.

Environmental conditions are also hypothesized to drive the evolution of different shapes between the sexes. Evidence for one environmentally-driven hypothesis is presented in a study looking at environmental gradients underlying SD and parallel evolution of a species of guppy *Poecilia reticulata* [28]. Results indicate that populations experiencing high predation were made up of males with smaller heads and deeper caudal peduncles. Open canopy sites resulted in selection for females with smaller heads and distended abdomens, whereas both sexes in high flow sites had small heads and deeper caudal peduncles. Males and females showed some shared responses to the environmental gradients, thus indicating that environmental variables may be responsible for sexual shape dimorphism more than sexual selection pressures might be. More support for the hypothesis that environmental processes drive variation in sexual shape dimorphism is found in the Greater Antillean *Anolis* lizards that exhibit sexual size and shape dimorphism. Males and females use habitats differently and although sexual size dimorphism is not highly related to habitat use, sexual shape dimorphism is [77]. Further study on West Indian *Anolis* lizards also suggests environment as a major factor driving the patterns of sexual shape dimorphism. Concordant with the Greater Antillean *Anolis* lizards, the shape dimorphism clearly reflects the different niches occupied by males and females [43].

Although these and numerous other examples demonstrate the influence of environment on the evolution of sexual shape dimorphism, a recent study examined sexual shape dimorphism in the snapping turtle *Chelydra serpentina*, and found no evidence that environmental condition was correlated with shape dimorphism. Unlike sexual size dimorphism, shape dimorphism was evident at hatching and at 15.5 months, where both males and females exhibited this pattern under optimal and suboptimal conditions. When adults however, sexual size dimorphism was present and differed under conditions such that there is increased plasticity of the larger sex as compared to the smaller. Interestingly however, sexual shape dimorphism still did not vary with differing conditions [57]. It has been suggested for over a century that environment is a major driver of morphological differences [78, 79], and new evidence such as this presents an opportunity to further understand the variables at play in the evolution of shape dimorphism.

Broadly, allometry (defined as a change in shape related to a change in size: 45) has also been suggested as having an influential impact on sexual shape dimorphism [80, 81]. In an example of evolutionary allometry, Gidaszewski *et al.* [45] examined sexual shape dimorphism in the wings of nine species of *Drosophila melanogaster* in a phylogenetic framework. Sexual shape dimorphism diverged among the nine species, however the evolution of sexual shape dimorphism was constrained by evolutionary history. This provides evidence that, while allometry is a large part of the evolution of sexual shape dimorphism in this system, it is not the main factor driving shape dimorphism.

Kaliontzopoulou *et al.* [82] studied heterochronic patterns of allometry in two species of lizard, *Podarcis bocagei* and *P. carbonelli*. Here, allometry did influence sexual shape dimorphism such that males and females actually differed in allometry with respect to head shape and body size, where change in male size increased disproportionately relative to head size and dimensions. Yet another recent study on sexual shape dimorphism in the stalk-eyed fly *Teleopsis dalmanni* found conclusive evidence for the impact of allometry on sexual shape dimorphism, where the size of the eye bulbs decreased with an increasing eye span and eyestalks became more elongated as they became thinner (Figure 7; 83).

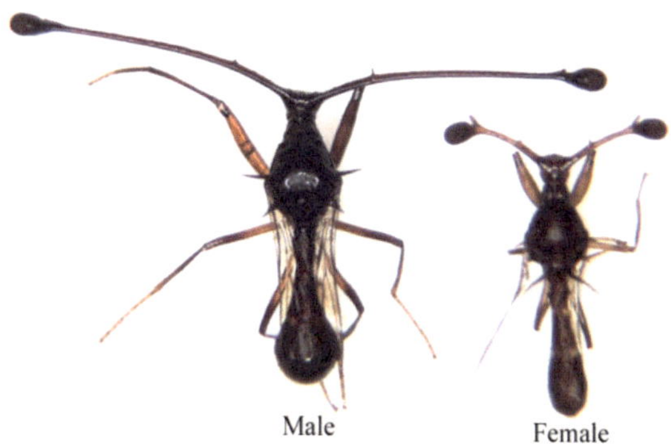

Figure 7. Sexual shape dimorphism in eye stalks of *Teleopsis dalmanni* (Photo credit: Jerry Husak)

Exceptions continue to be found however. For instance, in a recent study examining sexual size and shape dimorphism in the bill morphology of two hummingbirds *Archilochus colubris* and *A. alexandri*, Berns and Adams [58] examined a model that included an allometric component. This model was found to be inferior to those that included size, shape, and sex. When graphically depicted, it was clear that allometry is a less influential factor in the evolution of sexual shape dimorphism. However, as shown by the studies above it seems that allometry is generally an important process driving the patterns of evolution in sexual shape dimorphism.

Conserved genetics may be yet another factor driving patterns of sexual shape dimorphism. Sexual shape dimorphism has been studied in the piophilid fly *Prochyliza xanthostoma* (Piophilidae) and the neriid fly *Telostylinus angusticollis* (Neriidae) to address the impact of conserved genetic factors on patterns of sexual shape dimorphism [84]. These related species share similar patterns of sexual shape dimorphism, but have drastically different ecological and functional requirements as well as male-female interactions. Given that shape dimorphism is the similar trait in these three species, these flies may have congruent patterns of shape variation interspecifically, not due to common life-history requirements [84]. Bonduriansky suggests that this may be due to conserved genetics common to both species, or a reflection of interspecific variation in selection. In 2007, Bonduriansky [85] performed another study on *Telostylinus angusticollis* to examine condition-dependence and genetic variation. Sexual dimorphism is significantly correlated with the condition such that these two traits share a common genetic (and developmental) base. Therefore, it is possible that in this, as well as other systems, sexual shape dimorphism is a pleiotropic effect where sex-linked genes determine the allocation of traits differently in males and females. Any variation of these genes due to plasticity may then determine the genetic relationship of sexual shape dimorphism and differing conditions. Many genetic hypotheses continue to examine sexual size dimorphism and just recently is sexual shape dimorphism receiving attention.

4. Conclusion

Although studies are currently underway, many questions about sexual shape dimorphism still remain. For instance, how frequently is sexual shape dimorphism exhibited and how is this related to ontogenetic and biomechanical influences? Worthington *et al.* [83] propose that the sexually dimorphic patterns seen in the stalk-eyed fly are due to sexual selection, but also to biomechanical and possibly ontogenetic constraints. However, more information is necessary before a conclusion can be made about the actual process underlying the pattern of sexual shape dimorphism. Kaliontzopoulou *et al.* [82] suggest that a lack of sexual differences in cranial development of *Podarcis* species may indicate an ontogenetic limitation on both sexes, but also note that the habitat appears free of head constraint. The examination of ontogenetic development as well as biomechanical constraints on sexual shape dimorphism may reveal much about the causes and selective forces of these patterns, many of which are still unknown.

Does sexual shape dimorphism follow well-known patterns of sexual size dimorphism, such as Rensch's Rule? How much impact does allometry have in driving the evolution of sexual shape dimorphism? Although patterns such as these have been suggested as a component of sexual shape dimorphism, only recently have researchers begun to investigate these patterns. Is allometry in sexual shape dimorphism common? Berns and Adams [58] did not find a significant effect of allometry, whereas Worthington *et al.* did [83]. In species of *Drosophila melanogaster*, allometry did not explain the majority of evolutionary divergence of sexual shape dimorphism [45], while in *Podarcis bocagei* and *P. carbonelli,* Kaliontzopoulou *et al.* [82] showed that allometry was present and even differed in males and females. These inconcordant results suggest that there is a multifaceted interaction between sexual size dimorphism, sexual shape dimorphism and allometry. Examining size alone shows only a piece of the mechanisms contributing to allometry, thus attention needs to also focus on allometry and it's relationship with sexual shape dimorphism.

As seen in the examples in this chapter, much of the evidence on processes underlying sexual shape dimorphism is incongruent. One area needing attention is that of the correlation between sexual shape dimorphism and fecundity advantage, as shape may impact egg carrying capacity as size does. More work is needed to assess genetics and sexual shape dimorphism, and studies continue to argue that sexual selection causes sexual shape dimorphism due to male-male combat and mate choice, while others argue for natural selection via environmental factors and interspecific competition. No doubt that all of these factors play a role in influencing the evolution of sexual shape dimorphism, but what are the patterns? Do vertebrates tend to follow one trend while invertebrates follow another? In closely related species, does body size impact the effect of condition dependent sexual shape dimorphism? Just how much can natural selection and sexual selection be teased apart?

We are just beginning to test the questions about the role evolutionary history plays in patterns of sexual shape dimorphism. How do phylogenetic relationships effect sexual shape dimorphism? What role does sexual shape dimorphism play in microevolutionary patterns and what are the mechanisms underlying these patterns? What might result when these patterns are scaled from micro- to macroevolution? One way to address these questions is to take a sequential comparative approach: first examining patterns of dimorphism in two closely related species, then scaling up to family, genera, and so forth. It is now also possible to ask if rates of evolution differ between species and if these rates differ more broadly between different sexually dimorphic traits. What effect do habitat and environmental gradients play in assessing rates and patterns of sexual shape dimorphism evolution? By examining the possible correlation between sexual shape dimorphism and habitat variables in a phylogenetic manner, it is possible to quantify hypotheses such as these. With the advent of new phylogenetic techniques, morphometric methods, and statistical testing, we can further examine the details of the evolution of sexual shape dimorphism.

Author details

Chelsea M. Berns
Department of Ecology, Evolution and Organismal Biology, Iowa State University, Ames, Iowa, USA

Acknowledgement

I would like to thank D. C. Adams, A. Alejandrino, J. P. Chong, A. Kaliontzopoulou and C. P. Ceballos for comments on this chapter. I also thank the United States National Science Foundation for financial support through the Graduate Research Fellowship DGE0751279.

5. References

[1] Stuart–Fox DM, Ord TJ. Sexual selection, natural selection and the evolution of dimorphic coloration and ornamentation in agamid lizards. Proceedings of the Royal Society of London Series B: Biological Sciences. 2004;271(1554):2249-55.
[2] Endler JA. Natural and sexual selection on color patterns in poeciliid fishes. Environmental Biology of Fishes. 1983;9(2):173-90.
[3] Moore AJ. The Evolution of Sexual Dimorphism by Sexual Selection: The Separate Effects of Intrasexual Selection and Intersexual Selection.
[4] Watson NL, Simmons LW. Mate choice in the dung beetle Onthophagus sagittarius: are female horns ornaments? Behavioral Ecology. 2010;21(2):424-30.
[5] Geist V, Bayer M. Sexual dimorphism in the Cervidae and its relation to habitat. Journal of Zoology. 2009;214(1):45-53.

[6] Loyau A, Saint Jalme M, Cagniant C, Sorci G. Multiple sexual advertisements honestly reflect health status in peacocks Behavioral Ecology and Sociobiology. 2005;58:552-7.
[7] Ananjeva NB, Tsellarius AY. On the factors determining desert lizards' diet. In: Rocek(ed.) IZ, editor. Studies in Herpetology. Charles University, Prague1986. p. 445-8.
[8] Stiles FG. Time, energy, and territoriality of the Anna Hummingbird (*Calypte anna*). Science. 1971;173(3999):818-21.
[9] Armstrong DP. Economics of breeding territoriality in male Calliope Hummingbirds. The Auk. 1987;104(2):242-53.
[10] Shine R. Sexual size dimorphism and male combat in snakes. Biomedical and Life Sciences. 1978;33(3):269-77.
[11] Ralls K. Sexual Dimorphism in Mammals: Avian Models and Unanswered Questions.
[12] Hedrick AV, Temeles EJ. The evolution of sexual dimorphism in animals: hypotheses and tests. Trends in Ecology & Evolution. 1989;4(5):136.
[13] Abouheif E, Fairbairn DJ. A comparative analysis of allometry for sexual size dimorphism: assessing Rensch's Rule. The American Naturalist. 1997;149(3):540-62.
[14] Andersson M. Sexual Selection. Princeton University Press P, NJ, editor: Princeton University Press, Princeton, NJ; 1994.
[15] Darwin CR. The Descent of Man and Selection in Relation to Sex. London: John Murray; 1871.
[16] Jones AD, Ratterman NL. In the Light of Evolution III: Two Centuries of Darwin Sackler Colloquium: Mate choice and sexual selection: What have we learned since Darwin? Proceedings of the National Academy of Sciences. 2009.
[17] Stuart-Fox D. A test of Rensch's rule in dwarf chameleons (Bradypodion spp.), a group with female-biased sexual size dimorphism. Evolutionary Ecology. 2009;23(3):425-33.
[18] Bean D, Cook JM. Male mating tactics and lethal combat in the nonpollinating fig wasp Sycoscapter australis. Animal Behavior. 2001;62:535-42.
[19] Weatherhead PJ, Robertson RJ. Offspring quality and the polygyny threshold: "The Sexy Son Hypothesis". The American Naturalist. 1979;113(2):201-8.
[20] Hunt J, Breuker CJ, Sadowski JA, Moore AJ. Male–male competition, female mate choice and their interaction: determining total sexual selection.
[21] Fisher RA. The evolution of sexual preference. The Eugenics Review. 1915;7(3):184-92.
[22] Fisher RA. The Genetical Theory of Natural Selection. Oxford: Clarendon Press; 1930.
[23] G. EW. Sexual Selection and Animal Genitalia. Cambridge, MA: Harvard University Press; 1985.
[24] Selander RK. Sexual selection and dimorphism in birds. Sexual Selection and the Descent of Man (1871-1971): Aldine, Chicago, IL; 1972. p. 180-230.
[25] Slatkin M. Ecological Causes of Sexual Dimorphism. Evolution. 1984;38:622-30.
[26] Shine R. Ecological Causes for the Evolution of Sexual Dimorphism: A Review of the Evidence. Quarterly Review of Biology. 1989;64:419-61.
[27] Butler MA, Schoener TW, Losos JB. The relationship between sexual size dimorphism and habitat use in Greater Antillean *Anolis* lizards. Evolution. 2000;54:259-72.

[28] Hendry AP, Kelly ML, Kinnison MT, Reznick DL. Parallel evolution of the sexes? Effects of predation and habitat features on the size and shape of guppies. J Evol Biol. 2006;19:741-54.

[29] Lovich JE, Gibbons JW. A review of techniques for quantifying sexual size dimorphism. Growth, development, and aging : GDA. 1992;56(4):269-81.

[30] Stephens PR, Wiens JJ. Evolution of sexual size dimorphisms in Emydid turtles: Ecological dimorphism, Rensch's Rule, and sympatric divergence. Evolution. 2009;63(4):910-25.

[31] Rensch B. Die Abha ̈ngigkeit der relativen Sexualdiffer- enz von der Ko ̈rpergro ̈sse. Bonn Zool Beitr 1950;1:58-69.

[32] Fairbairn DJ, and, Preziosi RF. Sexual selection and the evolution of allometry for sexual size dimorphism in the water strider, *Aquarius remigis*. The American Naturalist. 1994;144(1):101-18.

[33] Fairbairn DJ. Allometry for sexual size dimorphism: Pattern and process in the coevolution of body size in males and females. Annual Review of Ecology and Systematics. 1997;28(1):659-87.

[34] Williams GC. Adaptation and natural selection: Princeton University Press, Princeton, NJ; 1966.

[35] Hughes AL, Hughes MK. Paternal investment and sexual size dimorphism in North American passerines. Oikos. 1986;46:171-5.

[36] Colwell RK. Rensch's Rule crosses the line: convergent allometry of sexual size dimorphism in hummingbirds and flower mites. The American Naturalist. 2000;156(5):495-510.

[37] Berry JF, Shine R. Sexual size dimorphism and sexual selection in turtles (order testudines). Oecologia. 1980;44(4):185-91.

[38] Young KA. Life–history variation and allometry for sexual size dimorphism in Pacific salmon and trout. Proceedings of the Royal Society B: Biological Sciences. 2005;272:167-72.

[39] Székely. T, Freckleton RPa, Reynolds RJ. Sexual selection explains Rensch's rule of size dimorphism in shorebirds. Proceedings of the Academy of Sciences of Philadelphia. 2004;101(33):12224-7.

[40] Fairbairn DJ. Allometry for sexual size dimorphism: Testing two hypotheses for Rensch's rule in the water strider *Aquarius remigis*. American Naturalist. 2005;166(4):S69-S84.

[41] Blanckenhorn WU, Stillwell RC, Young KA, Fox CW, Ashton KG. When Rensch meets Bergmann: does sexual size dimorphism change systematically with latitude? Evolution. 2006;50:2004-11.

[42] Hendry AP, Grant PR, Grant BR, Ford HA, Brewer MJ, Podos J. Possible human impacts on adaptive radiation: beak size bimodality in Darwin's finches. Proceedings of the Royal Society B-Biological Sciences. 2006;273(1596):1887-94.

[43] Butler MA, Sawyer SA, Losos JB. Sexual dimorphism and adaptive radiation in *Anolis* lizards. Nature. 2007;447:202-5.

[44] Lande R, Arnold SJ. Evolution of mating preference and sexual dimorphism. Journal of Theoretical Biology. 1985;117(4):651.

[45] Gidaszewski NA, Baylac M, Klingenberg CP. Evolution of sexual dimorphism of wing shape in the *Drosophila melanogaster* subgroup. BMC Evolutionary Biology. 2009;9:110.

[46] Berns, CB, Adams, DC. Becoming different but staying alike: Patterns of sexual size and shape dimorphism in bills of hummingbirds. Evolutionary Biology. 2012; in press. DOI 10.1007/s11692-012-9206-3.

[47] Bookstein FL. Morphometric tools for landmark data: geometry and biology. Cambridge: Cambridge University Press; 1991.

[48] Dryden IL, Mardia KV. Statistical shape analysis. New York: John Wiley and Sons; 1998.

[49] Adams DC, Rohlf FJ, Slice DE. Geometric morphometrics: ten years of progress following the 'revolution'. Italian Journal of Zoology. 2004;71:5-16.

[50] Bookstein F, Schäfer K, Prossinger H, Seidler H, Fieder M, Stringer C, et al. Comparing frontal cranial profiles in archaic and modern Homo by morphometric analysis. The Anatomical Record. 1999;257(6):217-24.

[51] Slice DE. Modern morphometrics in physical anthropology: Kluwer Academic Publishers; 2005.

[52] Dryden IL, Mardia KV. Multivariate Shape Analysis. SankhyÄ: The Indian Journal of Statistics, Series A (1961-2002). 1993;55(3):460-80.

[53] Rohlf FJ. Shape statistics: Procrustes superimpositions and tangent spaces. J Classif. 1999;16:197-223.

[54] Adams DC, West ME, Collyer ML. Location-specific sympatric morphological divergence as a possible response to species interactions in West Virginia Plethodon salamander communities. Journal of Animal Ecology. 2007;76(2):289-95.

[55] Adams DC, Nistri A. Ontogenetic convergence and evolution of foot morphology in European cave salamanders (Family: Plethodontidae). BMC Evolutionary Biology. 2010;10:216.

[56] Adams DC. Parallel evolution of character displacement driven by competitive selection in terrestrial salamanders. BMC Evolutionary Biology. 2010;10:72.

[57] Herler J, Kerschbaumer M, Mitteroecker P, Postl L, Sturmbauer C. Sexual dimorphism and population divergence in the Lake Tanganyika cichlid fish genus *Tropheus*. Frontiers in Zoology. 2012;7(4).

[58] Ceballos CP, and, Valenzuela N. The role of sex-specific plasticity in shaping sexual dimorphism in a long-lived vertebrate, the snapping turtle *Chelydra serpentina*. Evolutionary Biology. 2011;38:163-81.

[59] Berns CM, Adams DC. Bill shape and sexual shape dimorphism between two species of temperature hummingbirds: *Archilochus alexandri* (black-chinned hummingbirds) and *Archilochus colubris* (ruby-throated hummingbirds). The Auk. 2010;127:626-35.

[60] Temeles EJ, Goldman RS, Kudla AU, Stouffer PC. Foraging and territory economics of sexually dimorphic Purple-throated Caribs (*Eulampis jugularis*) on three *Heliconia* morphs. The Auk. 2005;122(1):187-204.

[61] Berns CM, Adams DC. Becoming different but staying alike: patterns of sexual size and shape dimorphism in bills of hummingbirds. Evolutionary Biology. 2012;*In review*.

[62] Navarro J, Kaliontzopoulou A, Gonza'lez-Solıs J. Sexual dimorphism in bill morphology and feeding ecology in Cory's shearwater (*Calonectris diomedea*). Zoology. 2009;112:128-38.

[63] Kaliontzopoulou A, Carretero MA, Llorente GA. Intraspecific ecomorphological variation: linear and geometric morphometrics reveal habitat-related patterns within *Podarcis bocagei* wall lizards. Journal of Evolutionary Biology. 2010;23:1234-44.

[64] Kuo C-Y, Lin Y-T, Lin Y-S. Sexual size and shape dimorphism in an Agamid lizard, *Japalura swinhonis* (Squamata: Lacertilia: Agamidae). Zoological Studies. 2009;48(3):351-61.

[65] Vincent SE, Herrel A, Irschick DJ. Sexual dimorphism in head shape and diet in the cottonmouth snake (*Agkistrodon piscivorus*). Journal of Zoology, London. 2004;264:53-9.

[66] Herrel A, Schaerlaeken V, Moravec J, Ross CF. Sexual shape dimorphism in tuatara. Copeia. 2009;4:727-31.

[67] Herrel A, Moore JA, Bredeweg EM, Nelson NJ. Sexual dimorphism, body size, bite force and male mating success in tuatara. Biological Journal of the Linnean Society. 2010;100:287-92.

[68] Temeles EJ, Miller JS, Rifkin JL. Evolution of sexual dimorphism in bill size and shape of hermit hummingbirds (Phaethornithinae): a role for ecological causation. Philosophical Transactions of the Royal Society B: Biological Sciences. 2010;365(1543):1053-63.

[69] Temeles EJ, Pan IL, Brennan JL, Horwitt JN. Evidence for ecological causation of sexual dimorphism in a hummingbird. Science. 2000;289(5478):441-3.

[70] Temeles EJ, Kress WJ. Adaptation in a plant-hummingbird association. Science. 2003;300(5619):630-3.

[71] Monnet JM, Cherry MI. Sexual size dimorphism in anurans. Proceedings of the Royal Society B. 2002;269:2301-7.

[72] Tague RG. Big-bodied males help us recognize that females have big pelvis. American Journal of Physical Anthropology. 2005;127:392-405.

[73] Schwarzkopf L. Sexual dimorphism in body shape without sexual dimorphism in body size in water skinks (*Eulamprus quoyii*). Herpetologica. 2005;61:116-23.

[74] Olsson M, Shine R, Wapstra E, Ujvari B, Madsen T. Sexual dimorphism in lizard body shape: The roles of sexual selection and fecundity selection. Evolution. 2002;56(7):1538-42.

[75] Bonnet X, Lagarde F, Henen BT, Corbin J, Nagy KA, Naulleau G. Sexual dimorphism in steppe tortoises (*Testudo horsfieldii*): Influence of the environment and sexual selection on body shape and mobility. Biological Journal of the Linnean Society. 2001;72(3):357-72.

[76] Malmgren JC, Thollesson M. Sexual size and shape dimorphism in two species of newts, *Triturus cristatus* and *T. vulgaris* (Caudata: Salamandridae). Journal of Zoology, London. 1999;249:127-36.

[77] Willemsen RE, Hailey A. Sexual dimorphism of body size and shell shape in European tortoises. Journal of Zoology, London. 2003;260:353-65.

[78] Butler MA, Losos JB. Multivariate sexual dimorphism, sexual selection, and adaptation in the Greater Antillean *Anolis* lizards. Ecological Monographs. 2002;72(4):541-59.

[79] Darwin CR. On the origin of species by means of natural selection. London: John Murray; 1859.

[80] Grant PR, Grant BR. Adaptive radiation of Darwin's finches. American Scientist. 2002;90:130-9.

[81] O'Higgins P, Collard M. Sexual dimorphism and facial growth in papionin monkeys. Journal of Zoology, London. 2002;257:255-72.

[82] Schaefer K, Mitteroecker P, Gunz P, Bernhard M, Bookstein FL. Craniofacial sexual dimorphism patterns and allometry among extant hominids. Annals of Anatomy. 2004:471-8.

[83] Kaliontzopoulou A, Carretero MA, Llorente GA. Head shape allometry and proximate causes of head sexual dimorphism in *Podarcis* lizards: joining linear and geometric morphometrics. Biological Journal of the Linnean Society. 2008;93:111-24.

[84] Worthington AM, Berns CM, Swallow JG. Size matters, but so does shape: quantifying complex shape changes in a sexually selected trait in stalk-eyed flies (Diptera: Diopsidae). Biological Journal of the Linnean Society. 2012;106:104-13.

[85] Bonduriansky R. Convergent evolution of sexual shape dimorphism in Diptera. Journal of Morphology. 2006;267:602-11.

[86] Bonduriansky R. The evolution of condition-dependent sexual dimorphism. The American Naturalist. 2007;169(1):9-19.

Chapter 2

Sexual Dimorphism in Antennae of Mexican Species of *Phyllophaga* (Coleoptera: Scarabaeoidea: Melolonthidae)

Angel Alonso Romero-López and Miguel Angel Morón

Additional information is available at the end of the chapter

http://dx.doi.org/10.5772/55313

1. Introduction

Sexual dimorphism in body, antennae, lamellae and chemosensilla types of some Mexican species of *Phyllophaga* are recorded. In *Phyllophaga obsoleta* and *Phyllophaga ravida* the male's body is slightly larger than the female's, and its antennae and lamellae are longer than the females. Meanwhile, in *Phyllophaga opaca* the body and its antennae and lamellae of the males are very similar in size than the females. The external morphology of sensilla on the antennae has been described using scanning electron microscopy. The antennal club of these beetles consists of three terminal plates: proximal, middle, and distal lamellae. In all these species, the main sensilla types were identified on the internal and external surfaces of lamellae from both sexes: placodea (PLAS), auricilica (AUS), basiconica (BAS), coeloconica (COS), trichodea (TRS), and chaetica (CHS). The first four types have been considered as chemosensilla and the last two as mechanoreceptor sensilla. For *P. opaca*, fifteen types of chemosensilla were found: four types of PLAS (I, II, III and VIII), four types of AUS (I, II, III and IV), five types of BAS (I, II, III, IV and V), and two types of COS (I and III). This is very similar to that observed in *P. ravida* and therefore it is suggested that these data can relate to the taxonomy of the genus *Phyllophaga*, since both species belong to the same subgenus. To give continuity to this type of comparative studies with other Mexican species of Melolonthidae to complement the information on the phylogeny of the group, is necessary in addition to their chemical communication, information about their sexual dimorphism phocused on antennal micro-morphology, genital structure, and reproductive behavior.

2. Sexual dimorphism in Coleoptera

Outstanding structural differences between males and females of many species of beetles have been described by naturalist and scientists during the last 200 years. Most part of such differences is located on the head and prothorax of males, such as in the form and size of the mandibles, length of antennal or palpi segments, horn-like structures on the frons or on the pronotal surface. Other differences are found in the size of whole body, development of elytra and hind wings, as well as in the length of fore and hind legs, or in the shape of pygidial plate. Less frequent is the strong difference in color or body vestiture. Flightless females are commonly found in species of many families, but larval-like females are the rule into the species of Phengodidae [1,2,3,4]. Sexual dimorphism is more common in the species of the suborder Polyphaga than in the suborder Adephaga, and appears to be a recent feature, because few fossil specimens of diverse families dated from Pliocene and Pleistocene shown dimorphic structures [5,6,7].

3. Sexual dimorphism in Coleoptera Scarabaeoidea

"A most remarkable distinction between the sexes of many beetles is presented by the great horns which rise from the head, thorax and clypeus of the males... These horns, in the great family of Lamellicorns, resemble those of various quadrupeds, such as stags, rhinoceroses, etc. and are wonderful both from their size and diversified shapes. … The females generally exhibit rudiments of the horns in the form of small knobs or ridges; but some are destitute of even a rudiment…. The extraordinary size of the horns, and their widely different structure in closely-allied forms, indicate that they have been formed for some important purpose; but their excessive variability in the males of the same species leads to the inference that this purpose cannot be of a definite nature. … The most obvious conjecture is that they are used by the males for fighting together; but they never had been observed to fight…" [8].

Members of the superfamily Scarabaeoidea (Lamellicornia and Pectinicornia) exhibit ones of the most striking dimorphic structures of the beetle species. Cephalic horn-like projections are present in the males of species from the subfamilies Dynastinae, Rutelinae, Cetoniinae, Scarabaeinae, and Geotrupinae. Much enlarged mandibles are common in the males of the subfamilies Lucaninae, Dorcinae, Lampriminae, Chiasognathinae and Odontolabinae. Males of Melolonthinae, Rutelinae and Pleocomidae frequently show the segments of the antennal club enlarged and expanded. Pronotal horn-like or tooth-like projections are developed in the males of the subfamilies Dynastinae, Cetoniinae, Scarabaeinae, Geotrupinae and Orphninae. Much enlarged fore legs (femur, tibia, tarsus) are characteristic in males of the subfamily Euchirinae, meanwhile males of the genus *Pachylomera* (Scarabaeinae) have fore femora much swell. Enlarged hind legs (femur and tibia) are observed in males of some genera of Rutelinae and Scarabaeinae. Females apterous or with short hind wings have been reported in nearly all the subfamilies of Scarabaeoidea, but the female of *Pachypus candidae* Petagna (Pachypodinae) lacks also the elytra. Except for horn-like structures, usually, males have smaller and slender bodies than females, but females of the family Pleocomidae are much larger and stouter than males [9,10].

3.1. Dimorphism and behavior in Melolonthidae (chafers, rhinoceros beetles)

Following the classification of [11] updated by [12], the family Melolonthidae ("melolonthids") is formed by the world wide members of Melolonthinae (sensu lato),

Rutelinae and Dynastinae. Some species of these subfamilies are famous by it striking sexual differences. First example, each antenna of the male of *Polyphylla petiti* Guerín (Melolonthinae) is formed by seven enlarged, flattened antennomeres that are five times longer than the remainder three basal antennomeres, meanwhile each antenna of the female is formed by five briefly elongated antennomeres that are as long as the remainder five antennomeres. It is evident that the much expanded olfactory surface of the male is developed in correspondence with the perception of sex compounds produced by the female [13].

Second example, metasternum of the male of *Chrysina macropus* Francillon (Rutelinae) strongly produced, hind coxa is wide, hind femur is swollen and provided with a strong spine, and the tibia is enlarged and curved with setae on the inner border (Figures 1 A-B), in the female the metasternum is flattened, hind coxa and femur are much narrower than in male and hind tibia is short and nearly straight, without setae on the inner border. Looks like the male embraces female with his large hind legs during coupling, but really these legs are not used in this form. It is much possible that are useful during combat with other co-specific males as forceps formed between femur and tibia, that may produce much force derived from the increased musculature inside the metathorax, coxa and femur; such forceps also may be used as defense against big predators [Morón unpublished data].

Third example, horn-like projections on the head and pronotum of *Dynastes hercules* L. (Dynastinae) may be as long as body length or even longer that this. Both projections may act as long forceps, applying force derived from cervical muscles to head projection. Such force is sufficient to cut or broken the elytra of other male of "Hercules beetle", but is useful to embrace it a turnout of the tree branches where they inhabit, after fighting during some minutes. But this conclusion needed many years to mature, because much speculation surrounded the observation of dead specimens in collections, and studies of live beetles in nature or in captivity were scarce and incomplete during near a century. After a long discussion on the dimorphic structures in horned beetles, with arguments and data of other authors, including Darwin, [14] concluded that "The horns of a beetle, the size of which is increasing gradually as generations succeed one another, will as a result become more and more disproportionate in size, regardless of the fact that they may be quite useless, and the absence of the restraining and modeling influence of natural selection will be a contributory cause of the acquisition of fantastic forms."

A large number of observations on captive Hercules beetles in Venezuela support the following comments: "The sequence of the beetle encounter is unvarying. The two meet head on, and the projecting horns touch and click, spread wide and close, the whole object of the opening phase being to get a grip outside the opponent's horns. When the four horns are closed together, there is a deadlock. All force in now given to pinching, with the apparent desire to crush and injure some part of head or thorax. Again and again, both opponents back away, freeing their weapons, and then rush in for a fresh grip. Once this hold is attained and a firm grip secured, the beetle rears up and up to an unbelievably vertical stance. At the zenith of this pose it rests upon the tip of the abdomen and the tarsi of

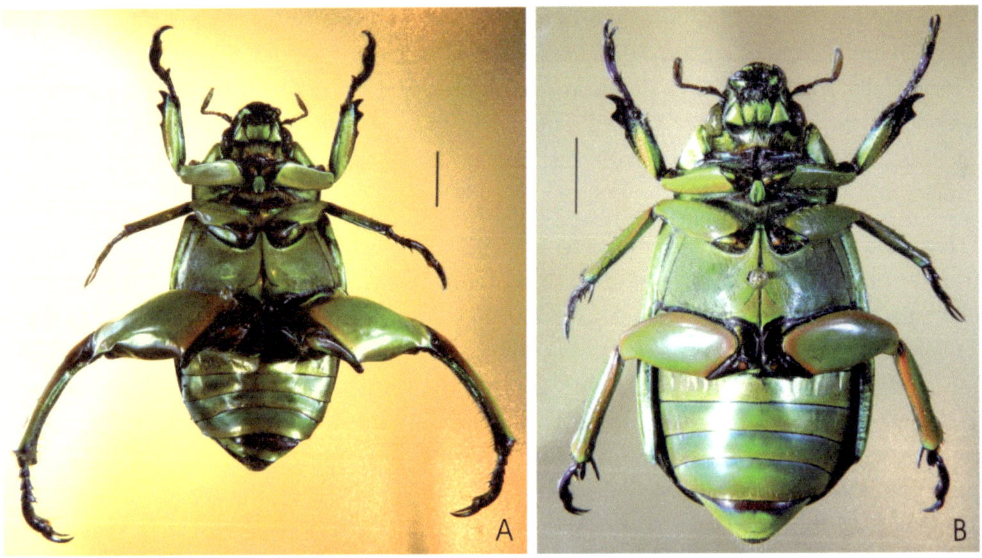

Figure 1. *Chrysina macropus* Francillon. (A) Male, ventral view, showing the hypertrophied hind legs. (B) Female, ventral view. Scale lines 5 mm. Photos M. A. Morón.

the hind legs, the remaining four legs outstretched in mid air, and the opponent held sideways, kicking impotently… after 2-8 seconds the victim is slammed down or is carried away … before to banging to earth will take place" [15]. Other academics discussed on the essential components of such phenomenon or on details of the above described behavior, as [16] who comments: "The display of species showing extreme intrasexual selection function both to attract females to intimidate other males. Precopulatory displays are short or absent. The male Hercules beetle, for example, evidently engages in none whatever. Occasionally he picks a female up and carries her aimlessly about for a short while, but the significance of the behavior is unknown. During both transportation and copulation the female remains outwardly passive". With elegance and precision, [17] objectively wrote: "The only function for beetle horns which has been confirmed by detailed observations is that of weapons for use in intraspecific fights. Many horn designs remain to be studied… More data are needed to answer outstanding questions about the significance of multiple horn designs and the selective pressures favoring fighting in some species. Several factors may have predisposed beetles to evolve horns more readily than other insects".

3.2. Study of dimorphism in melolonthid beetles in Mexico

The males of nearly all the species of Melolonthidae usually present a number of small structural differences more or less directly associated with the search of females and coupling behavior. Most of these modifications are located in the legs, as tarsal pads, specially curved tarsal claws, tibial spurs, rows of tarsal setae, etc. Other modifications are developed on the last sternites and pygidial plate [18]. Many of these are frequently applied as taxonomic characters, but it function remain generalized. Few studies on the allometric growth of hypertelic structures in species with strong sexual dimorphism had been published in Mexico [19,20].

Scarce research had been carried on the microstructures, mainly on those related with sensorial functions, as the diverse types of sensilla placed on the lamellar surfaces of antennomeres such as was detailed by [21]. These structures were briefly studied in some Mexican species by [18,22,23,24]. The structure, distribution and function of the antennal sensilla reveal much interest, because represent the main way to understand the pre-reproductive behavior, and the evolution of the chemical communication in this group of insects.

4. Studies of sexual dimorphism in antennae of Mexican species of *Phyllophaga*

Sexual chemical communication in some Melolonthidae involves the production and release of specific chemicals by the emitter and the detection and olfactory processing of these signals leading to appropriate behavioral responses in the receiver [25]. Chemicals released from melolonthid females are captured in the sensilla located on both sides of male antennal lamellae [21,18,26]. The genus *Phyllophaga* is formed by more than 800 species, but only in *Phyllophaga anxia* LeConte [27] and in the antennae of Mexican species *Phyllophaga obsoleta* Blanchard [23] and *Phyllophaga ravida* Blanchard [24] have the different types of sensilla been studied. In the following sections data from *P. obsoleta* and *P. ravida* are remembered and compared with the data of another species of *Phyllophaga* distributed in Mexico.

4.1. Methodology for the study of antennae of Mexican melolonthids

4.1.1. Measurement of body, antennae and lamellae dimensions

After taxonomical identification using the keys proposed by Morón [18], females and males of *P. obsoleta, P. ravida* and *Phyllophaga opaca* Moser were randomly chosen for length measurement with the Image Tool 3.0 software program [28]. Length was measured in each specimen from the clypeus to the pygidium. The head of each previously measured specimen was separated from the body and preserved in 70% ethanol. The antennae of females and males of each species were separated and measurements of total length, width, and area of each lamella, were obtained with the Image Tool 3.0 software program. Afterwards, the three lamellae forming each antennal club were separated, labeled, and grouped according to sex and lamellar side (internal or external surfaces). The lamella located farther away from the head was denominated distal lamella (DL), while the nearest was called proximal lamella (PL) and the one between these two, middle lamella (ML).

4.1.2. *Specimen preparation for light microscopy studies*

Antennae from females and males of each species were kept in 10% KOH at 80ºC for 60 min, rinsed in distilled water, and placed in 70% ethanol in order to separate the lamellae, which were then dehydrated in 80%, 90%, and absolute ethanol. Lamellae were placed in xylene during 10 min for clearing, mounted in Canadian balsam and observed under a light microscope (Iroscope, Mod. MG-11J). Images from these slides and from non-cleared lamellae were obtained with a photo-microscope III (Carl Zeiss) and a Tessovar microscope (Carl Zeiss), both including a PaxCam 3 digital camera.

4.1.3. *Specimen preparation for scanning electron microscopy studies*

Lamellae from additional specimens were prepared following the methods proposed by [29] and were examined at 25kV under a scanning electron microscope (JEOL Mod. JSM-5600LV).

4.1.4. *Statistics*

Data on body, antennae and lamellae dimension for *P. opaca, P. ravida* and *P. obsoleta,* and adult males and females were analyzed with Student's t or Mann-Whitney Rank Sum tests (SigmaStat 3.1; 3.5). Unless otherwise stated, all values reported are mean ± standard error.

5. Sexual dimorphism in antennae of *Phyllophaga obsoleta*

This is one of the most noxious *Phyllophaga* species in México [30]. *Phyllophaga obsoleta* female's body length is larger than males, but the lamellar club is significantly longer and wider in males than females (Figures 2 A-B, Table 1). In males, PL and ML were longer and had a larger area than in females (Table 1). Also, DL in males were longer, had a larger area and greater width than in females (Table 1).

Classification and terminology of sensilla types used here are based principally on [31] and in part on [21,32,27]. Six types of sensilla in both surfaces of antennal lamellae of both sexes of *P. obsoleta* were identified: sensilla placodea (PLAS), sensilla auricilica (AUS), sensilla basiconica (BAS), sensilla coeloconica (COS), sensilla trichodea (TRS) and sensilla chaetica (CHS). In Figure 3, these different sensilla types are showed. PLAS are thin-walled plates or are low dome shaped and BAS are cone-shaped. AUS are characterized by a "rabbit-ear" shape. COS are rarely found as aggregations of long rods located inside cuticle cavities. COS are observed only on internal surfaces of all lamellae from both sexes. TRS have a long hair-like structure that occurs along the peripheral edges while CHS present a short-bristle- or spine-like structure; they occur along the peripheral edges and some are in the lamellar center. According with above cited authors, TRS and CHS types are most likely mechano-receptors, but PLAS, AUS, BAS, and COS are considered chemo-receptor types.

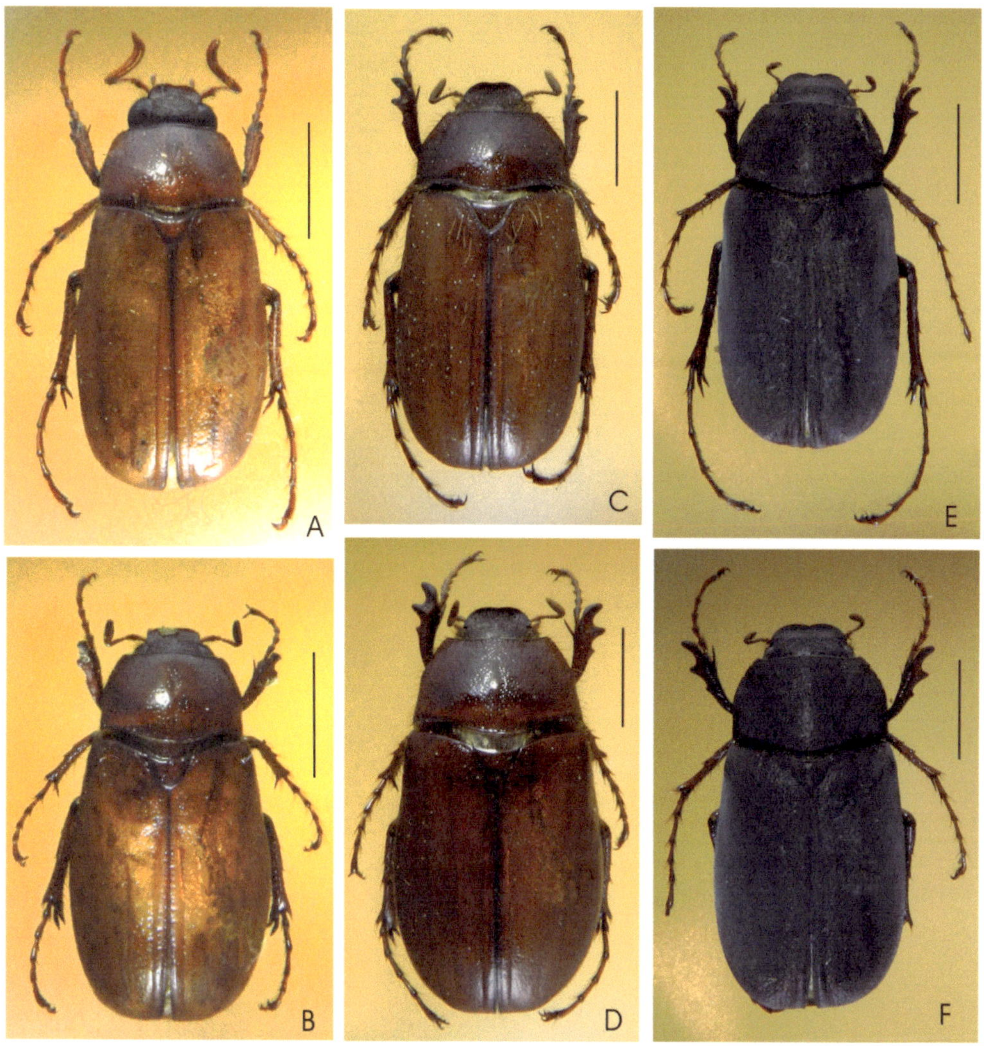

Figure 2. Habitus of species of *Phyllophaga*. *Phyllophaga obsoleta,* (A) male; (B) female. *Phyllophaga ravida,* (C) male; (D) female. *Phyllophaga opaca,* (E) male; (F) female. Scale lines 5 mm. Photos M. A. Morón.

		POBS			*PRAV*			*POP*	
	F	M	*p*	F*	M*	*p*	F**	M**	*p*
MEASURE (*mm*)									
Body	18.18 ±0.3	17.19 ±0.2	<0.05	22.13 ±0.3	21.17 ±0.2	<0.05	22.12 ± 0.2	21.16 ± 0.5	*0*
Entire antennae	3.30 ± 0.08	3.90 ± 0.04	<0.001	3.37 ±0.02	4.07 ±0.05	<0.001	2.88 ± 0.03	3.08 ± 0.05	<0.001
Antennal flagellum	2.15 ± 0.08	2.20 ± 0.04	*0*	0.99 ±0.01	1.06 ±0.01	<0.05	1.80 ± 0.03	1.98 ± 0.04	<0.001
Antennal club	1.15 ± 0.02	1.70 ± 0.02	<0.001	1.15 ±0.01	1.71 ±0.02	<0.001	1.09 ± 0.01	1.10 ± 0.01	*0*
PL length	1.07 ± 0.02	1.66 ± 0.04	<0.001	1.19 ± 0.01	1.71 ± 0.04	<0.001	0.92 ± 0.02	0.95 ± 0.02	<0.05
PL area (mm²)	0.28 ± 0.01	0.51± 0.02	<0.001	0.38 ± 0.01	0.63 ± 0.02	<0.001	0.25 ± 0.01	0.26 ± 0.01	*0*
PL width	0.35 ± 0.01	0.38 ± 0.01	*0*	0.41 ± 0.01	0.46 ± 0.01	<0.05	0.35 ± 0.01	0.36 ± 0.01	*0*
ML length	1.10 ± 0.02	1.60 ± 0.03	<0.001	1.13 ± 0.01	1.67 ± 0.03	<0.001 (1)	0.81 ± 0.01	0.90 ± 0.02	<0.001
ML area (mm²)	0.29 ± 0.03	0.48 ± 0.04	<0.001	0.36 ± 0.01	0.61 ± 0.02	<0.001	0.19 ± 0.01	0.22 ± 0.01	<0.05
ML width	0.36 ± 0.01	0.37 ± 0.01	*0*	0.41 ± 0.01	0.47 ± 0.01	<0.05	0.30 ± 0.01	0.32 ± 0.01	<0.05
DL length	1.04 ± 0.03	1.58 ± 0.04	<0.001	1.04 ± 0.01	1.60 ± 0.03	<0.001	0.69 ± 0.02	0.82 ± 0.01	<0.001
DL area (mm²)	0.23 ± 0.01	0.44 ± 0.01	<0.001	0.31 ± 0.01	0.54 ± 0.01	<0.001	0.13 ± 0.02	0.17 ± 0.01	<0.001
DL width	0.31 ± 0.01	0.37 ± 0.01	<0.001	0.38 ± 0.01	0.42 ± 0.01	<0.001	0.24 ± 0.01	0.27 ± 0.01	<0.05

Values are mean ± standard error of the mean; *Student t*-test; *0*= not significant; (1)= Mann-Whitney Rank Sum test
POBS: Phyllophaga obsoleta, n= 12; PRAV: Phyllophaga ravida, n= 14; POP: Phyllophaga opaca, n= 13; F= females; M= males; * n=20; **= n=6; PL = proximal lamella; ML = middle lamella; DL = distal lamella

Table 1. Comparison of the body and antennae dimensions, length, width and area of the lamellae of females and males of *Phyllophaga obsoleta, Phyllophaga ravida and Phyllophaga opaca.*

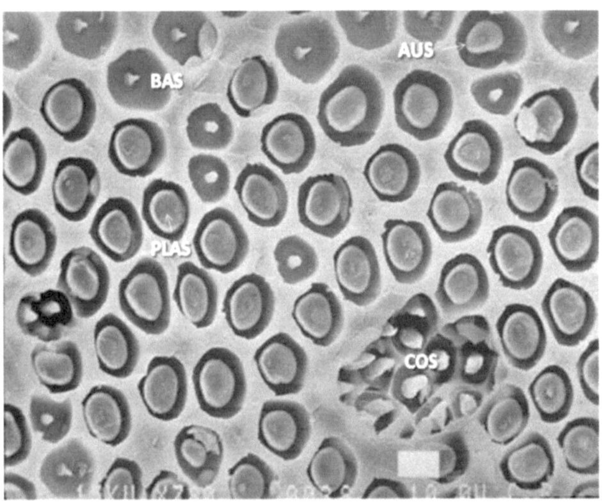

Figure 3. Scanning electron-micrograph of the internal surface (IN) of male *Phyllophaga obsoleta* middle lamella (ML). The IN is almost entirely covered by four sensillar types. In the periphery of the lamella, TRS and CHS are observed. B) TRS (long hair or setae shape). C) CHS (spine shape). D) PLAS (thin-walled plate or low dome), BAS (cone- or rod-shape) and AUS ("rabbit-ear-like") on the IN of the ML. E) Another view of PLAS, BAS and AUS. F) PLAS, BAS, AUS and COS (long rod aggregations located inside cuticle cavities). G) Detail of PLAS, BAS and COS. Micrographies by J. Valdez.

6. Sexual dimorphism in antennae of *Phyllophaga ravida*

Phyllophaga ravida is included in the "*dentex*" complex of the "*ravida*" species group, subgenus *Phyllophaga* (*sensu stricto*), and is one of the main white grub species of agricultural and economic importance in Mexico [30]. Several sex-related differences in antennae are observed. Although the body of adult *P. ravida* females is larger than that of males, the entire male antenna is considerably longer (Figures 2 C-D, Table 1). In males, DL is longer, wider, and cover a larger area than in females. Furthermore, the male ML is longer, with a larger area and greater width. Finally, male PL is longer, with a larger area and greater width (Table 1). Several types of sensilla were observed on *P. ravida* antennae using light- and scanning electron-microscopy: PLAS, AUS, BAS, COS, TRS and CHS (Table 2). TRS have a long spine- or hair-like structure and CHS present a short-spine, being shorter than TRS (Table 2). For *P. ravida*, sixteen chemo-sensilla types were found: three types of PLAS, four of AUS, five of BAS, and four of COS.

Morphological characteristics of each chemo-sensilla type are described in the Table 2.

Sensilla types	Morphological characteristics
PLAS I	large spherical plates
PLAS II	spherical or elliptical and thin-walled plates
PLAS III	small and elliptical thin-walled plates or low dome-shaped plates
AUS I	elliptical and thin walled-plates with "rabbit-ear" shape
AUS II	small "rabbit-ear" shaped structures, elliptical and low dome-shaped
AUS III	"human-ear" shaped structures
AUS IV	small "rabbit-ear with neck" or "raisin with neck" shaped structures
BAS I	large peg- or cone-shaped
BAS II	short-spine shaped
BAS III	short peg- or cone shaped
BAS IV	serrated-cone shaped
BAS V	long-rod shaped
COS I	aggregations of 2 to 16 long peg- or cone-shaped structures (BAS I)
COS II	aggregations of 2 to 3 serrated cone-shaped structures (BAS IV)
COS III	long, rod-shaped aggregations (BAS V)
COS IV	aggregations of a long cone (BAS I) and a spherical plate (PLAS I)
TRS	long hair-like structure
CHS	short-bristle- or spine-like structure

PLAS= sensilla placodea; AUS= sensilla auricilica; BAS= sensilla basiconica; COS= sensilla coeloconica; TRS= sensilla trichodea; CHS= sensilla chaetica.

PLAS, AUS, BAS and COS are present on internal surface of lamellae while TRS and CHS are structures that occurs along the peripheral edges of each lamella and some are in the lamellar center.

Table 2. Morphological description of each of the types of antennal sensilla observed in the lamellae of males or females of *Phyllophaga ravida*.

For both sexes, PLAS type I were observed randomly distributed on internal surface (IN) of all lamellae mainly in the center, except on peripheral edges of lamellae. PLAS type II were observed randomly distributed on IN and at the peripheral edges of all lamellae in both male and females. PLAS type III were located on IN of all lamellae, principally on pit, basal, and peripheral edges in both sexes. AUS type I were observed randomly distributed on IN and peripheral edges of all lamellae for both sexes. AUS type II was observed only in male lamellae, distributed on both sides (except on the external surface of the DL). AUS type III was located only on male lamellae, randomly distributed on IN and on peripheral edges (except on the IN of DL). AUS type IV were restricted to the center of PL in males. BAS type I were observed randomly distributed mostly on IN of all club lamellae of both sexes (except on peripheral edges and on the IN of ML). BAS type II are present for both sexes, they are situated on IN and peripheral edges of all lamellae. For both sexes, BAS type III were observed randomly distributed principally on IN of all club lamellae, except on peripheral edges. BAS type IV were found only in females at the center of the IN of ML and PL. BAS type V were found only in males, mainly at the center of the IN of PL. For both sexes, COS type I are restricted principally to the center, appearing only at the IN of all club lamellae. COS type II are located in both sexes, on the floor of cuticle cavities. COS type II are restricted only to females, mostly at the center and only on the IN of all club lamellae, except on DL. COS type III are located inside cavities in the antennal cuticle. COS III are restricted principally to the center, appearing only on the IN of all club lamellae in both sexes, except on male PL. COS type IV are found only in males and are restricted to the center and IN of PL. They are located inside depressions or cavities in the antennal cuticle.

7. Sexual dimorphism in antennae of *Phyllophaga opaca*

Phyllophaga opaca is distributed in the states of Michoacan and Sinaloa, Mexico [30]. Some general characteristics of its flight and eating habits [33], the nature of its chemical sexual communication, and the structures involved in the production of its sex pheromone [25] are known, although there are no data regarding of its sexual dimorphism in body and antennae. Although the body of adult *P. opaca* males is very similar in size than the females, the entire male antenna is significantly longer (<0.001) (Figures 2 E-F, Table 1). In males, DL and ML were longer and had a larger area than in females (Table 1). Also, PL in males were longer than in females (Table 1).

PLAS, AUS, BAS, COS, TRS and CHS were observed on *P. opaca* antennae (females and males) using light- and scanning electron-microscopy (Figures 4 and 5). TRS have a long spine- or hair-like structure and CHS present a short-spine, being shorter than TRS (Table 2, Figure 4). For *P. opaca*, fifteen chemo-sensilla types were found: four types of PLAS, four of AUS, five of BAS, and two of COS.

For both sexes, PLAS type I were observed randomly distributed on IN of all lamellae mainly in the center, except on peripheral edges of lamellae; they are rounded and elongated plates (Figures 4C-D, Table 2). PLAS type II were observed in both males and females, randomly distributed on IN of all lamellae mainly in the center; they are spherical

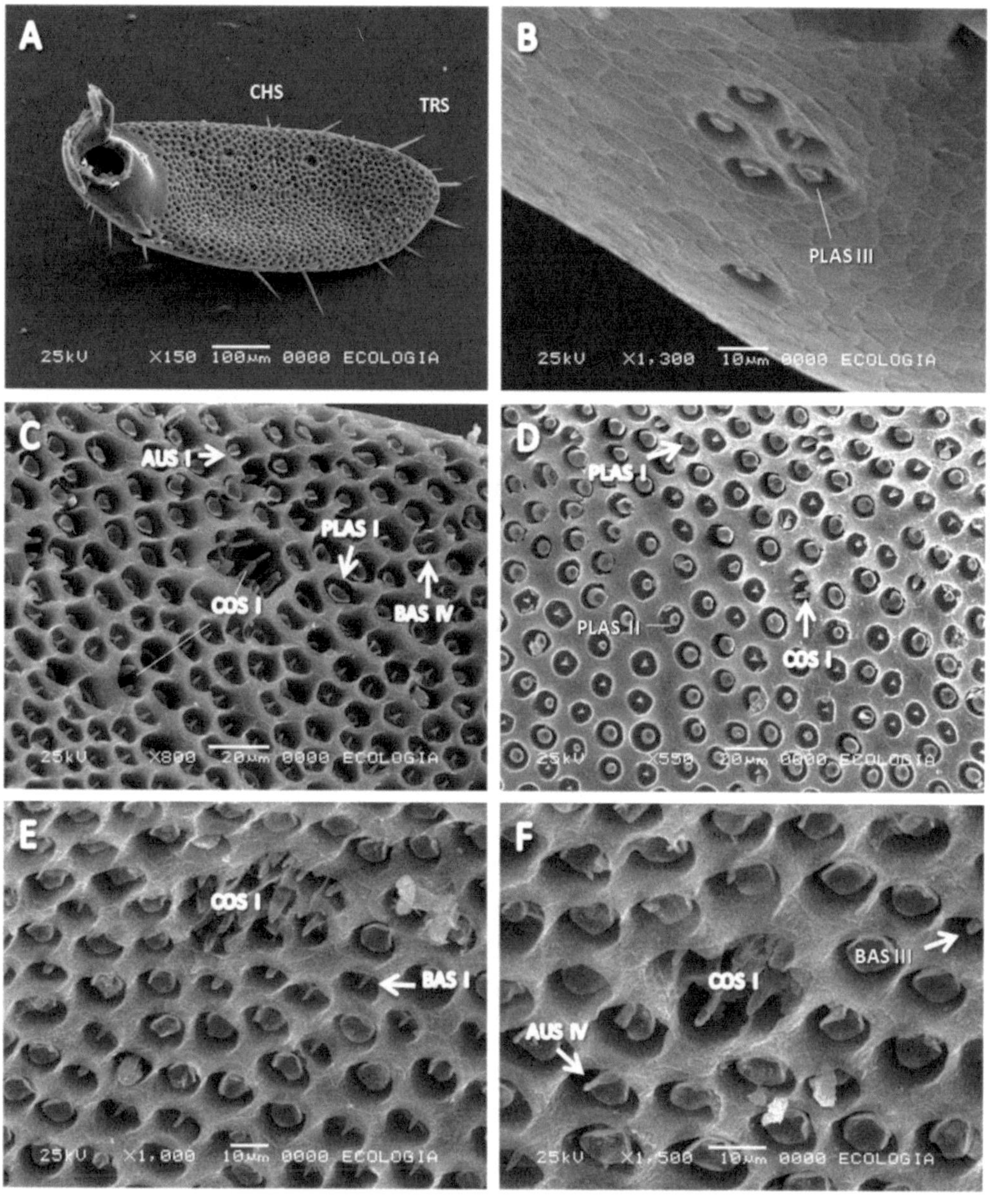

Figure 4. Sensilla on the antennae of female *Phyllophaga opaca*. A) Internal surface (IN) of distal lamella (DL). In the periphery of the lamella, trichodea (TRS) and chaetica sensillum (CHS) are observed. B) Detail of placodea sensilla (PLAS) type III on external (EX) of proximal lamella (PL). C) Coeloconica sensilla (COS) type I, auricilica sensilla (AUS) type I, basiconica sensilla (BAS) type IV and PLAS I on IN of DL. D) Detail of COS I, PLAS I y PLAS II on IN of medium lamella (ML). E) COS I and BAS I on IN of PL. F) Detail of COS I, AUS IV and BAS III on IN of PL. Micrographies by T. Laez.

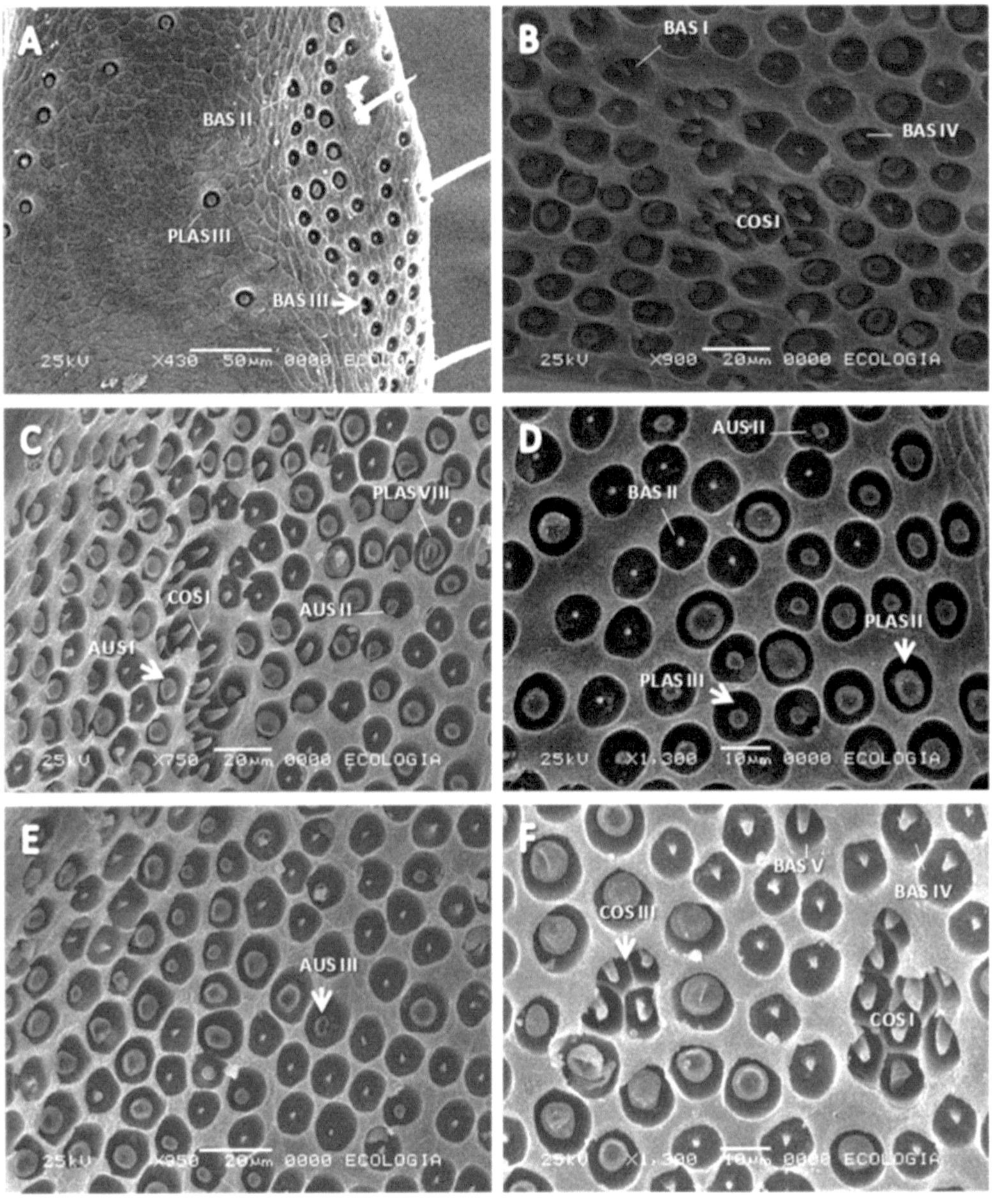

Figure 5. Sensilla on the antennae of male *Phyllophaga opaca*. A) External surface (EX) of proximal lamella (PL). Detail of placodea sensilla (PLAS) type III, basiconica sensilla (BAS) type II and III. B) Coeloconica sensilla (COS) type I, BAS I and BAS IV on internal surface (IN) of distal lamella (DL). C) Detail of auricilica sensilla (AUS) type I and II, COS I and PLAS VIII on IN of PL. D) PLAS II, PLAS III, AUS II and BAS II on IN of medium lamella (ML). E) Detail of AUS III on IN of PL. F) COS I, COS III, BAS IV and BAS V on IN of PL. Micrographies by T. Laez.

or elliptical and thin-walled plates (Figures 4D-5D, Table 2). PLAS type III are located on both sides of all lamellae, principally on pit and peripheral edges in both sexes; they are small, elliptical, thin-walled plates or low dome-shaped plates (Figures 4B-5A, Table 2). PLAS type VIII are chemoreceptors not reported previously; they are spherical or elliptical and thin-walled plates with "human-ear" like structure in the center. PLAS VIII were observed only in males lamellae, randomly distributed on IN of DL (Figure 5C).

AUS type I were observed randomly distributed on IN of all lamellae for both sexes; they are characterized by a "rabbit-ear" shape or elliptical and thin-walled plates (Figures 4C-5C, Table 2). AUS type II were observed only in male lamellae, distributed on IN of ML and DL; they are "rabbit-ear" shaped structures, elliptical and low dome-shaped (Figures 5C-D, Table 2). AUS type III were located only on male lamellae, randomly distributed on IN of lamella center (except on the IN of DL); they are characterized by a "human-ear" shape (Figures 5E, Table 2). AUS type IV were restricted to the center of PL in both sexes; their shape is characterized as "rabbit-ear with neck" or "raisin with neck" structures (Figure 4F, Table 2).

BAS type I were observed randomly distributed mostly on IN of all club lamellae of both sexes (except on peripheral edges and on the external surface of ML); they are large peg- or cone-shaped (Figures 4E-5B, Table 2). BAS type II are short-spine shaped; for both sexes, they are situated on both sides of all lamellae (Figure 5D, Table 2). BAS type III were observed for both sexes distributed on both sides of all lamellae; they are short-cone shaped (Figures 4F-5A, Table 2). BAS type IV were found randomly distributed on IN of all club lamellae of both sexes of PL and DL; they are serrated-cone shaped (Figures 4C-5B-5F, Table 2). BAS type V were found only in males, mainly at the center of the IN of PL; they are long-rod shaped (Figure 5F, Table 2).

For both sexes, COS type I are restricted principally to the center, appearing only at the IN of all club lamellae. They are found as aggregations of 2 to 16 long peg- or cone-shaped structures (BAS I) located inside depressions or cavities in the antennal cuticle (Figures 4 and 5, Table 2). COS type II were found as aggregations of two to three serrated cone-shaped structures (BAS IV) located on the floor of cuticle cavities. These cavities vary in size between 11.58 and 17.54 μm on the largest axis. COS type III are restricted principally to the center, appearing only on IN of male PL (Figure 5F, Table 2).

8. Analysis between species - sexual dimorphism

As described in this chapter, in the melolonthids there is a marked sexual dimorphism at different levels. In the case of the members of the genus *Phyllophaga*, mainly for Mexican species have been studied some morphological traits that allow differentiate between females and males. For antennae, at least three species studied show sexual dimorphism in body size, length of the antennae and lamellae, and the presence/absence of certain types of sensilla. Sexual dimorphism in antennae of these species is evident when considering antennal/body length ratio. For *P. obsoleta* and *P. ravida* males, the length of the antennal club represent almost one fourth of the body length (Table 1). This is evident in the antennae of several melolonthid species, in which males have longer antennae than females [18,10,34,35]. Furthermore, sexual differences in antennal length are mostly evident in the lamellar club, which is the most important sensorial zone for pheromone and allelochemical perception for these insects [23]. Because *P. obsoleta, P. ravida* and *P. opaca* males have longer antennae, longer and wider lamellae, and greater antennal area, males can be regarded as the receptors in their sexual chemical communication [25]. Previous studies with these species have provided morphological and biological evidence that females display a calling behavior during which they expose the protractile genital chamber from the abdominal tip and release chemical compounds that are attractive to males [36,25].

In *P. opaca,* the size and proportions of antennae of male is nearly similar as in female, so may be hypothesised that olphactory sensilla works in different form or that sexual attractant is distinct. Functional olphactory antennal surface (club lamellar area) in male of *P. opaca* is two times smaller than in the antennae of *P. ravida,* and 1.5 times smaller than in the antennae of *P. obsoleta* (Table 1).

The morphological study for *P. opaca* receptors is the second for melolonthids with several different types of antennal sensilla (after the *P. ravida* record). In similar studies, antennal

Sensilla types	*POBS*	*PRAV*	*POP*
PLAS I	X	X	X
PLAS II	X	X	X
PLAS III	X	X	X
AUS I	X	X	X
AUS II	X	X	X
AUS III		X	X
AUS IV		X	X
BAS I	X	X	X
BAS II	X	X	X
BAS III	X	X	X
BAS IV		X	
BAS V		X	
COS I	X	X	X
COS II		X	
COS III		X	X
COS IV		X	
TRS	X	X	X
CHS	X	X	X

PLAS= sensilla placodea; AUS= sensilla auricilica; BAS= sensilla basiconica; COS= sensilla coeloconica; TRS= sensilla trichodea; CHS= sensilla chaetica.

PLAS, AUS, BAS and COS are present on internal surface of lamellae while TRS and CHS are structures that occurs along the peripheral edges of each lamella and some are in the lamellar center.

POBS: Phyllophaga obsoleta

PRAV: Phyllophaga ravida

POP: Phyllophaga opaca

Table 3. Comparison of the different sensilla types of the lamellae of females and males of *Phyllophaga obsoleta, Phyllophaga ravida and Phyllophaga opaca.*

lamellae of other species have a maximum of six sensilla types [27,23,35]. For Coleoptera in general, only thirteen types of sensilla have been reported in three different Carabidae species [37]. Previous studies for others species use terminology and classification based largely on [21] and [31]; these papers report the main sensilla types as PLAS, BAS, and COS [34,38], including the AUS [27,23]. Part of the results obtained in *P. opaca* clearly show a distinct sexual dimorphism principally with PLAS VIII and COS III, observed only in males. The data obtained at the time allow viewing two main perspectives to continue with studies of this type: data useful in taxonomy and data that allow relating the morphology of the sensilla with the sexual behaviour of the Mexican species of *Phyllophaga*. On the one hand, we found evidence that the types of antennal receptors could be support some subgroups into the studied genus. For example, the main types of chemo-sensilla were presented in both *P. ravida* and *P. opaca* studied: PLAS I, PLAS II, PLAS III, AUS I, AUS II, AUS III, AUS IV, BAS I, BAS II, BAS III, COS I and COS III (Table 3), which belong to the subgenus *Phyllophaga*.

Phyllophaga obsoleta, P. ravida and *P. opaca* belongs to three of the groups of Mexican species proposed by [18,30]. During forcoming years we expect to study representative species of most of the remaining 38 groups, their sexual dimorphism, phocused on antennal micro-morphology, genital structure, production of chemical attractans and reproductive behavior.

Author details

Angel Alonso Romero-López
Escuela de Biología, Benemérita Universidad Autonóma de Puebla, Puebla, Mexico

Miguel Angel Morón
Instituto de Ecología, Xalapa, Veracruz, Apartado postal 63, Mexico

Acknowledgement

A. Aragón (BUAP) helped with collection of specimens of *P. ravida* and G. Lugo (UAS) with collection of specimens of *P. opaca*. A special thanks to J. Valdez (COLPOS) and T. Laez (INECOL) with scanning electron microscope images. A.A.R.L. is grateful to INECOL for financial support during his postdoctoral stay.

9. References

[1] Crowson RA. The biology of the Coleoptera. Academic Press: London 802 p; 1981.
[2] Lawrence JF. Order Coleoptera. In: Stehr FW (ed.) Immature Insects vol. 2. Kendall /Hunt Publishing Co. Dubuque: 1991. p144-658.
[3] Beutel RG, Leschen RAB. Morphology and systematics (Archostemata, Adephaga, Myxophaga, Polyphaga partim). Coleoptera, Beetles Vol. 1. Walter de Gruyter: Berlin 567 p; 2005.

[4] Leschen RAB, Beutel RG, Lawrence JF. Coleoptera, Beetles. Vol. 2 Morphology and systematics (Elateroidea, Bostrichiformia, Cucujiformia partim). De Gruyter: Berlin 786 p; 2010.

[5] Arnol'di LV, Zherikhin VV, Nikritin LM, Ponomarenko AG. Mesozoic Coleoptera. Oxonian Press Pvt. Ltd: New Delhi 285 p; 1991.

[6] Grimaldi D, Engel MS. Evolution of the insects. Cambridge University Press: New York 755 p; 2005.

[7] Krell FT. Fossil record and evolution of Scarabaeoidea (Coleoptera: Polyphaga). Coleopterists Society Monographs 2006; 5: 120-143.

[8] Darwin C. The descent of man. Chapter X. vol. II. John Murray: London. 406 p; 1871.

[9] Paulian R, Baraud J. Faune des Coléoptéres de France II Lucanoidea et Scarabaeoidea. Éditions Lechevalier: Paris 477 p; 1982.

[10] Morón MA. Escarabajos 200 millones de años de evolución. Instituto de Ecología AC y Sociedad Entomológica Aragonesa: Zaragoza 204 p; 2004.

[11] Endrödi S. 1966. Monographie der Dynastinae (Coleoptera Lamellicornia) I Teil. Entomologische Abhandlungen. Staatlichen Museum für Tierkunde in Dresden 1966; 33: 1- 457.

[12] Morón MA. Diversidad y distribución del complejo "gallina ciega" (Coleoptera: Scarabaeoidea). In: Rodríguez del Bosque LA, Morón MA (eds.). Plagas del suelo. Mundi-Prensa México: 2010a. p41-63.

[13] Morón MA. Las especies americanas de *Polyphylla* Harris (Coleoptera: Melolonthidae, Melolonthinae): biología e importancia agrícola. In: Rodríguez del Bosque LA, Morón MA (eds.). Ecología y control de plagas edafícolas. Instituto de Ecología AC México: 2010b. p1-17.

[14] Arrow GJ. Horned Beetles. A study of the fantastic in nature. Dr. W. Junk Publishers: The Hague 154 p; 1951.

[15] Beebe W. High jungle. Readers Union John Lane: London 234 p; 1952.

[16] Wilson EO. Sociobiology. The new synthesis. Belknap Press of Harvard University Press: Cambridge 697 p; 1975.

[17] Eberhard WG. The function of horns in *Podischnus agenor* (Dynastinae) and other beetles. In: Blum MS, Blum NA (eds.). Sexual selection and reproductive competition in insects. Academic Press Inc. New York: 1979. p231-258.

[18] Morón MA. El género *Phyllophaga* en México. Morfología, distribución y sistemática supraespecífica (Insecta: Coleoptera). Instituto de Ecología AC: México 341 p; 1986.

[19] Morón MA. Los estados inmaduros de *Inca clathrata sommeri* Westwood (Coleoptera. Melolonthidae, Trichiinae) con observaciones sobre el crecimiento alométrico del imago. Folia Entomológica Mexicana 1983; 56: 31-51.

[20] Morón MA. Los estados inmaduros de *Dynastes hyllus* Chevrolat (Coleoptera. Melolonthidae, Dynastinae) con observaciones sobre su biología y el crecimiento alométrico del imago. Folia Entomológica Mexicana 1987; 72: 33-74.

[21] Meinecke CC. Reichsensillen und Systematik der Lamelicornia (Insecta, Coleoptera). Zoomorphologie 1975; 82: 1-42.

[22] Carrillo-Ruiz H, Morón MA. Study on the phylogenetic relationships of the Hopliids (Coleoptera: Scarabaeoidea). Proceedings Entomological Society of Washington 2006; 108 (3): 619-638.
http://www.zin.ru/animalia/coleoptera/pdf/Moron_Hopliids_2006.pdf

[23] Romero-López AA, Arzuffi R, Valdez J, Morón MA, Castrejón F, Villalobos FJ. Sensory organs in the antennae of *Phyllophaga obsoleta* (Coleoptera: Melolonthidae). Annals Entomological Society of America 2004; 97(6): 1306-1312.
http://www.bioone.org/doi/pdf/10.1603/00138746(2004)097%5B1306:SOITAO%5D2.0.CO%3B2

[24] Romero-López AA, Morón MA, Valdez J. Sexual dimorphism in antennal receptors of *Phyllophaga ravida* Blanchard (Coleoptera: Scarabaeoidea: Melolonthidae). Neotropical Entomology 2010a; 39(6): 957-966. http://dx.doi.org/10.1590/S1519-566X2010000600018

[25] Romero-López AA, Arzuffi R, Morón MA. Comunicación química sexual. In: Rodríguez del Bosque LA, Morón MA (eds.). Plagas del suelo. Editorial Mundi-Prensa México: 2010b. p83-96.

[26] Leal WS. Chemical ecology of phytophagous scarab beetles. Annual Review of Entomology 1998; 43:39-61.
http://www.guaminsects.net/CRB/docs/Leal%201998%20chem%20ecol%20phytophagous%20scarab%20beetles.pdf

[27] Ochieng SA, Robbins PS, Roelofs WL, Baker TC. Sex pheromone reception in the scarab beetle *Phyllophaga anxia* (Col: Scarabaeidae). Annals of Entomological Society of America 2002; 95:97-102.
http://ento.psu.edu/directory/publications/129OchiengEtAl2002.pdf

[28] Wilcox D, Dove S, McDavid W, Greer DB. UTHSCSA Image Tool for Windows version 3.0. [CD-ROM]. The University of Texas Health Science Center in San Antonio. U.S.A; 2002.

[29] Bozzola JJ, Russell LD. Electron Microscopy, 2nd Edition. Jones & Bartlett Publishers, Inc. 1998.

[30] Morón MA. Diversidad, distribución e importancia de las especies de *Phyllophaga* Harris en México (Coleoptera: Melolonthidae). In: Aragón A, Morón MA, Marín-Jarillo A (eds.). Estudios sobre coleópteros del suelo en América Publicación especial de la BUAP Puebla México: 2003. p1-27.

[31] Schneider D. Insect antennae. Annual Review of Entomology 1964; 9: 103-122.
http://www.annualreviews.org/doi/abs/10.1146/annurev.en.09.010164.000535

[32] Zacharuk RY. Ultrastructure and function of insect chemosensilla. Annual Review of Entomology 1980; 25: 27-47.
http://www.annualreviews.org/doi/abs/10.1146/annurev.en.25.010180.000331

[33] Lugo GA, Aragón A, Reyes-Olivas A, Casillas P, Villegas-Cota JR, Morón MA. Alimentación de adultos de Coleoptera Scarabaeoidea en el norte de Sinaloa, México. In: Rodríguez del Bosque LA, Morón A (eds.). Ecología y control de plagas edafícolas. Publicación especial del INECOL México: 2010. p127-139.

[34] Kim JY, Leal WS. Ultrastructure of pheromone-detecting sensillum placodeum of the Japanese beetle, *Popillia japonica* (Coleoptera: Scarabaeidae). Arthropod Structure & Development 2000; 29: 121-128.
http://www.sciencedirect.com/science/article/pii/S1467803900000220

[35] Tanaka S, Yukuhiro F, Wakamura S. Sexual dimorphism in body dimensions and antennal sensilla in the white grub beetle, *Dasylepida ishigakiensis* (Coleoptera: Scarabaeidae). Applied Entomology and Zoology 2006; 41:455-461.
https://www.jstage.jst.go.jp/article/aez/41/3/41_3_455/_pdf

[36] Romero-López AA, Aragón A, Arzuffi R. Estudio comparativo del comportamiento sexual de cuatro especies de *Phyllophaga* (Coleoptera: Melolonthidae). In: Estrada EG, Equihua A, Luna C, Rosas-Acevedo JL (eds.). Entomología mexicana Vol. 6 Publicación especial de la Sociedad Mexicana de Entomología México: 2007. p275-281.

[37] Ploomi A, Merivee E, Rahi M, Bresciani J, Ravn HP, Luik A, Sammelselg V. Antennal sensilla in ground beetles (Coleoptera, Carabidae). Agronomy Research 2003; 1: 221-228. http://agronomy.emu.ee/

[38] Baker GT, Monroe WA Sensilla on the adult and larval antennae of *Cotinis nitida* (Coleoptera: Scarabaeidae). Microscopy and Microanalysis 2005; 11:170-171.
http://journals.cambridge.org/abstract_S1431927605500448

Chapter 3

Sexual Dimorphism Using Geometric Morphometric Approach

Hugo A. Benítez

Additional information is available at the end of the chapter

http://dx.doi.org/10.5772/55195

1. Introduction

Comparison of anatomical characters between organisms has been a core element in comparative biology for centuries. Historically, taxonomic classification and understanding of biological diversity have been based mainly on morphological descriptions [1]. In the early twentieth century, comparative biology entered a transition from the description field and quantitative science, where morphological analysis had a similar revolution of quantification [2]. Based on this quantitative mathematical revolution, the study of morphology has had an important emphasis by developing statistical shape analysis. This made possible the combination of multivariate statistical methods and new ways to visualize a structure [3,4].

In geometric morphometrics (GM), the shape is defined as "any geometric information that remains when the effects of translation, scaling and rotation are removed from an object"[5]. According to [6,7] two techniques have been described: Landmark and Outline methods. Landmark geometric morphometrics is currently the most used tool in sexual dimorphism studies, where equivalent and homologous specific points are fixed in the biological structure being studied. Whereas outliner GM reduces contour shape in a structure by means of points built and located in its boundaries [8-10]. These tools allow studying organism shape and also size, providing sound graphic analyses to quantify and visualize morphometric variation within and between organism samples.

One of the most interesting sources of phenotypic variation in animals and plants has been sexual dimorphism, the study of which continues to be an important area of research in evolutionary biology. Sexual differences in morphological characters are a common phenomenon in many animal taxa, and their most conspicuous aspect is body size [11]. The direction of these differences, that is whether males or females are larger, varies from one group to another [12]. Most of the morphological variations of insects are due to effects associated with the environment, either phenotypic responses (plasticity) or particularly those which act during ontogenetic development [13]. Females are generally larger than males, and this gives them adaptive advantages such as greater fecundity and better parental care [14,15]. However, in some species males are longer but have less relative mass e.g. [16], which implies that the determination of sexual dimorphism requires more complex measurement techniques related, for example, with geometric shape [17]. Sexual dimorphism is of interest in entomological studies since frequently the differences between sexes are not obvious or the individuals are very small; thus, finding discriminating characters allows easy determination of sexes.

Studies of *Ceroglossus chilensis* shape have discussed that sexual dimorphism is usually concentrated in two sections of body shape: in the abdominal section, where this dimorphism variation is associated with an adaptative character due to the presence of female eggs; and changes in the pronotal section associated with male-male competition due to variation in sexual ratio in populations [17,18]. Other studies have used geometric variation of wing shape in insects as the dimorphism character, where the integrated geometric variation of veins is differentiated between male and female [19].

The following chapter is a brief description of sexual dimorphism of shape in insects and its evaluation by using new morphological tools that provide a visualization of the geometric shape, besides a description in 2 insect orders about the way in which sexual dimorphism variations that are not easily observed may be distinguished in different populations.

2. Geometric morphometrics methodology

Morphometrics is the study of shape variation and its covariation with other variables. The development of its new properties, capable of capturing shape, renders this new morphology to be considered geometric, being its introduction received as a "revolution" for the morphological analysis realm [20]. Shape is mathematically defined as all the geometric features of an object except its size, position and orientation [4]. In other words, changes in size, position and orientation do not change the shape of an object. Most of the research efforts in geometric morphometrics have concentrated on landmark data. Morphological landmarks are points that can be located precisely on each specimen under study with a clear correspondence in a one-to-one manner from specimen to specimen [7,21]. There are several methods for the analysis of curves and outlines. Outlines can be analyzed using semi-landmarks, which are the points that fall at defined intervals along a curve between two landmarks [22]. Semilandmarks can be analyzed with Procrustes superimposition like ordinary landmarks. Another outline method is perhaps the oldest type of geometric morphometrics – Fourier analysis [23]. Fourier methods use sine and cosine harmonic functions to describe the positions of outline coordinates. Fourier analysis can be applied to 2D outlines [23,24] or 3D closed surfaces [25,26]. Eigenshape is a third method for the analysis of outlines or curves [27,28]. In eigenshape, the coordinate points of an outline or curve are converted to a phi function, which is a list of the angles from one point to the next one in the series. Outline methods have been criticized because their individual coordinate points are not biologically homologous to each other [29], but this issue is important only in cases where a one-to-one mapping between individual variables and biological homology is required.

The principal and most important analysis of geometric morphometrics is called Procrustes superimposition, where only the shape information is extracted and the other components of variation in size, position and orientation can be removed, while taking care not to alter shape in any step of the procedure [4,9,30]. The extra components of variation can be removed by rescaling the configurations to a standard size, shifting them to a standard position, and rotating them to a standard orientation (Figure 1). Moreover, since none of the steps has changed the shape of the configurations, the variation after the procedure is the complete shape variation.

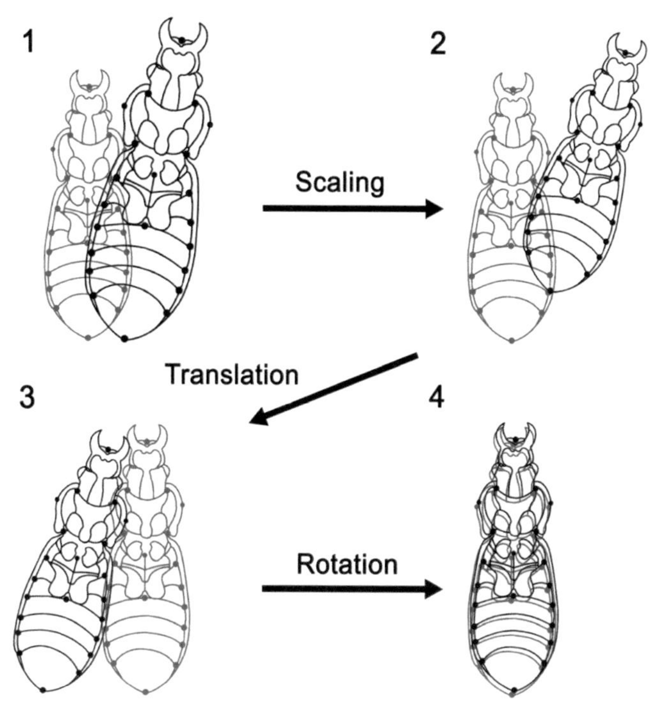

Figure 1. Summary of Procrustes superimposition. Components of variation other than shape are eliminated by scaling to the same size, translating to the same location of centroids, and rotating to an overall best fit of corresponding landmarks. (Figure Idea by C.P Klingenberg)

3. Sexual shape dimorphism

Insects in many species vary greatly in the expression of sexual traits [14]. In some species variation in the expression of such traits is discontinuous, resulting in the co-occurrence of two or more discrete phenotypes within one sex. The discrete expression of sexual traits or secondary sexual traits has attracted particular attention, as it is thought to reflect alternative adaptations to heterogeneous social conditions [31]. Sexual size dimorphism

(SSD) in body size is considered to be one of the major determinants of mating success in many species [32-35]. Because larger males are generally more aggressive and more competitive than smaller males, larger males often attain greater reproductive success through intrasexual selection [14]. In contrast, sexual shape dimorphism (SShD) has been much less investigated [17-19,36]. From those studies that considered SShD, most have discussed it as a diagnostic trait for diverse purposes, such as sex identification or the analysis of ontogeny [37-40]. Nevertheless, some other authors have considered sexual dimorphism evolution covering only some aspects of a limited number of taxa, such as: the evolution of cranium in primates [41-44]; the proportions and dimensions in lizard bodies [45,46]; newts [47]; or in flies [48]; and variation of shape in insect heads [49]; and variation of sexual dimorphism in *Drosophila* wings [36].

4. Sexual shape dimorphism examples in insect body and wing shape

4.1. Case 1 Body shape

In coleopteran of the genus *Ceroglossus* (Carabidae) a phenomenon occurs which is completely opposed to that described above. *Ceroglossus* Solier is a genus endemic to *Nothofagus* forests of the extreme south of South America.

Studies of body shape in *Ceroglossus chilensis* have demonstrated that the similarity of males and females is directly associated with the sex ratio of this species [50]. Morphological sex dimorphism is much reduced and only visible under a microscope. However, in terms of geometric morphometrics the differences are visible in two body regions; the abdomen of females, whose variation has been reported to have an adaptive value due to the presence of eggs, and changes in the pronotum of the thorax in males, which has been attributed to intrasexual competition in this species[17,18,50].

4.1.1. Methodology

For the morphometric analyses a total of 116 specimens of *C. chilensis* were used from 2 populations (53 males and 63 females) of Santa Juana area in the Coast Range (37º10'S, 72º57'W) and near San Fabián de Alico in the Andes Foothills (36º37' S, 71º50'W), both localities in the Región del Bío-Bío. The geometric analysis considered exclusively variation in shape, and it was performed using a photograph in ventral view of males and females with an Olympus X- 715 digital camera; using the methodology of [51], we digitized 17 landmarks (LMs, anatomical homologous points) on every picture, by TpsDig 2.10 (Figure 2). All analyses were then run using MorphoJ software version 1.05a [53].

Once the Cartesian x-y coordinates were obtained for all landmarks, the shape information was extracted with a full Procrustes fit [4,9], taking into account the object symmetry of the structure. Procrustes superimposition is a procedure that removes the information of size, position and orientation to standardize each specimen according to centroid size. Due to the high difficulty to check the differences in sexual dimorphism in this group, the only way to differentiate was based on the presence of antennal careens located from the fifth to ninth

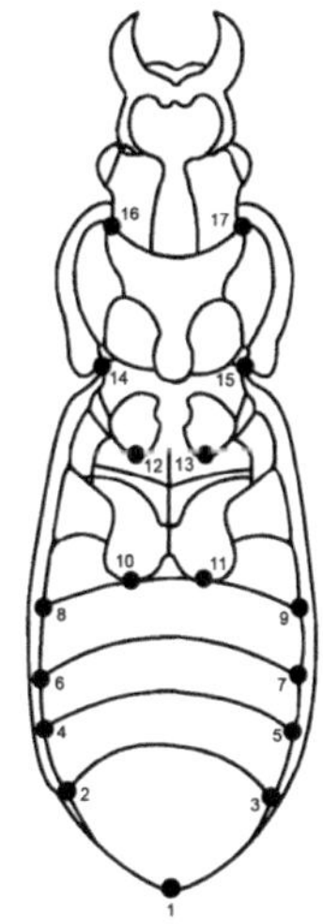

Figure 2. Location of the 17 landmarks in ventral view of *Ceroglossus chilensis*

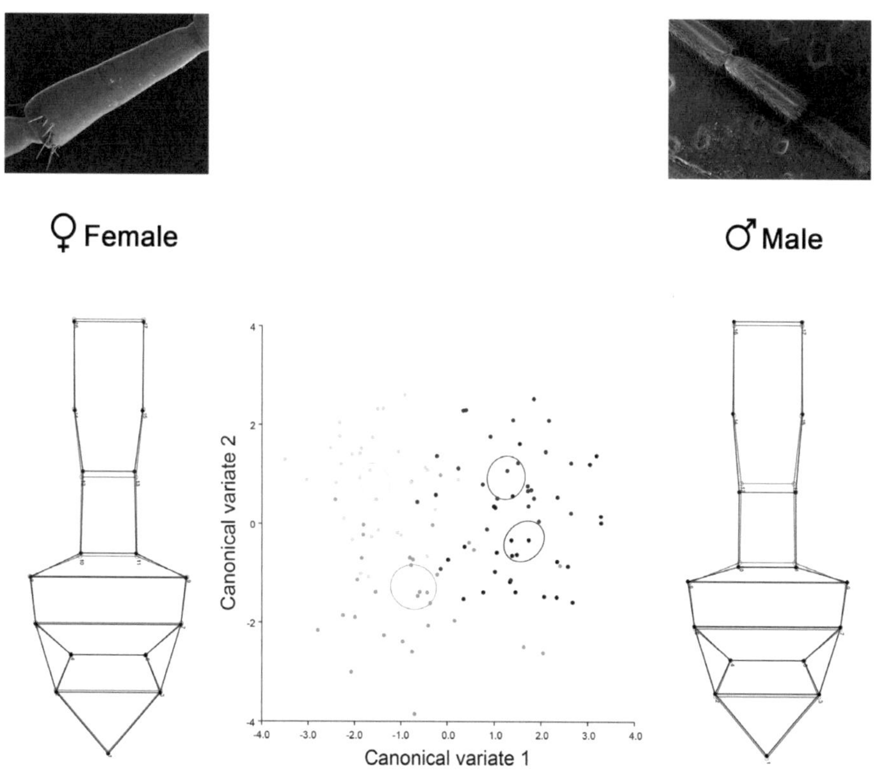

Figure 3. Canonical Variate Analysis (CVA) for the sexual shape dimorphism population of *Ceroglossus chilensis* *each point represents a shape variable for female and male individuals in ventral view. The figure shows the first two CV components' axes with shape deformation images associated, and their antennal structure that is differentiation characteristic based on optic microscopy (careens presence in males).

segment [54], present "only in males" and observable under a dissecting microscope (Figure 3). Because of the symmetry of the structure, reflection is removed by including the original and mirror image of all configurations in the analysis and simultaneously superimposing all of them [55]. To examine the amount of symmetric variation and sexual shape dimorphism we used Procrustes ANOVA to assess studies on object symmetry. Differences between locations and sex were assessed using canonical variate analysis (CVA), a multivariate statistical method used to find the shape characters that best distinguish multiple groups of specimens

4.1.2. Results

The PCA plot for the symmetric component (individual variation) shows some differences between the populations analyzed. The first two PCs account for 53.643% (PC1 + PC2 + PC3 = 27.619% + 14.88% + 11.14) of the total shape variation and provide a reasonable approximation of the total amount of variation, with the other PC components that account each no more than 9.5% of the variation. The canonic analysis showed a clear differentiation of sexual shape dimorphism in both populations (Figure 3).

The Procrustes ANOVA for size does not show significant differences between populations and sex. Instead, Procrustes ANOVA for shape shows differences between populations ($F = 3.79$, $P<0.0001$) and high differences between sex ($F = 11.76$, $P<0.0001$). Besides, MANOVA tests, for both symmetric and asymmetric components, confirm these results (Pillay = 0.64, $P<0.0001$; Pillay = 0.31, $P<0.0001$ respectively).

4.2. Case 2 Wing shape

Within species, sexual dimorphism is a source of variation in life history (e.g., sexual size dimorphism and protandry), morphology (e.g., wing shape and colour pattern), and behaviour (e.g., chemical and visual signaling). Sexual selection and mating systems have been considered the primary forces driving the evolution of sexual dimorphism in insects especially in lepidoptera, and alternative hypotheses have been neglected [56]. Recent analyses demonstrate that many lepidopteran species exhibit female-biased sexual size dimorphism 73% of 48 species in Reference [57]. Size and shape differences are established during the larval period [58,59] by developmental and physiological mechanisms (e.g., number of larval instars and hormonal regulation). Because females of many species are capital breeders (i.e., they allocate larval resources for reproduction), and large size is related directly to fecundity [60-62], selection for large female body size appears to be driven by natural selection for increased fecundity [63]. Most of the morphological variations between males and females in moth and buterflies are due to the effects associated with the environment, whether phenotypic responses (plasticity) or particularly those which act during ontogenetic development [64-66]. Females are generally larger than males; this gives them adaptive advantages such as greater fecundity and better parental care [14,15,63,67].

In this section, sexual dimorphism was determined to be present in the wing shape of moths of the *Synneuria* genus, suggesting that the wing shape may be selected as a character to determine sex between lepidopteran species.

4.2.1. Methodology

Sampling: The study area was the farms named "El Guindo (36º50'12''W- 73º01'25''S) and Coyanmahuida" (36°49'28.66"S - 72°44'1.34"W) separated 20 km from one another in the province of Concepción, Biobío Region of Chile, where there are relict native forests with *Nothofagus obliqua* and *Peumus boldus*, among others. In order to determine intra- and interpopulation variation by means of geometric morphometrics, we used adults of *Synneuria* sp. (Lepidoptera, Geometridae). The individuals were collected by phototropic UV traps using an 800 watt electric generator; the light sources were placed over a white sheet to increase the luminosity. These traps were installed for a period of 4 hours in different sampling points. Finally we collected individuals which were processed, males and females separated, wings cut, and mounted.

The geometrical analysis, which considered variations attributed exclusively to shape, was performed using a photographic register of 63 males and 58 females of *Synneuria* sp., whose wings were each mounted in a fixed mould. The right wing of each was photographed with a Sony 10 DSC-H7 camera with directed fibre optics lighting, with which we constructed photographic matrixes using the TpsUtil 1.40 program [68]. We digitalized 18 morphological landmarks based upon the shape and vein pattern of the wing (Figure 4) for all individuals using the TpsDig 2.12 program (52). To determine if there are significant differences between male and female populations of *Synneuria*, a factorial variance analysis (ANOVA) was calculated base on the matrix of covariance between sexes generated by means of the Procustes analysis.

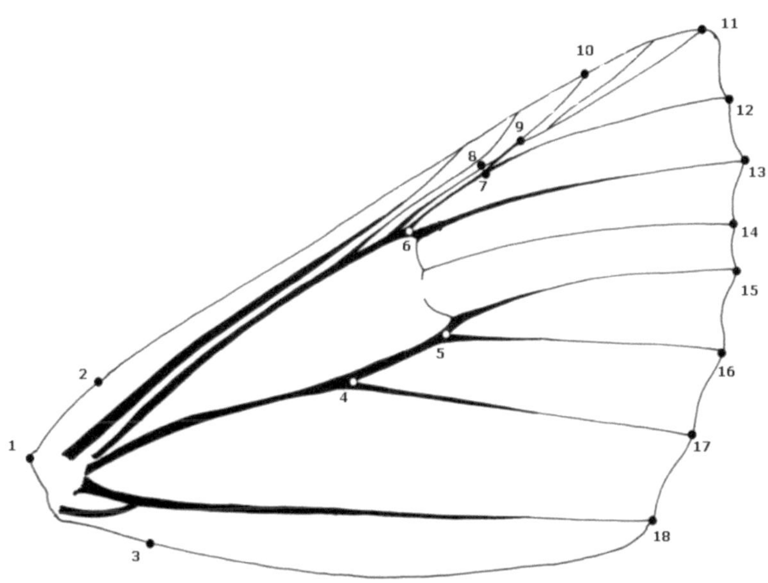

Figure 4. Location of 18 morphological landmarks in the right wing of *Syneuria* sp. (Benitez, Neotropical Entomology unpublished data)

4.2.2. Results

The morphological variation among moths determined by Procrustes ANOVA indicates that variation in shape between sexes is highly significant (Table 1).

Effect	SS	df	MS	F	p
Sex	**0.001526**	**1**	**0.001526**	**4.237204**	**0.018961**
Locality	0.000061	1	0.000061	0.169012	0.684121
Sex x Locality	0.000490	1	0.000490	1.360991	0.253206
Error	0.010086	28	0.000360		

Table 1. Two-way ANOVA for differences in shape of *Synneuria* sp using the first relative warp as dependent variable.

The relative warp plot shows some differences between sexes within each population analyzed (Figure 5). The first three Rws account for 91.74% of the total shape variation and provide a reasonable approximation of the total amount of variation, and the other Rw components account each for no more than 5% of variation. In order to visualize the variation in wing shape graphically we took the mean of the first three relative warps. We found different morphotypes for males and females of Coyanmahuida and Guindo (Figure 6).

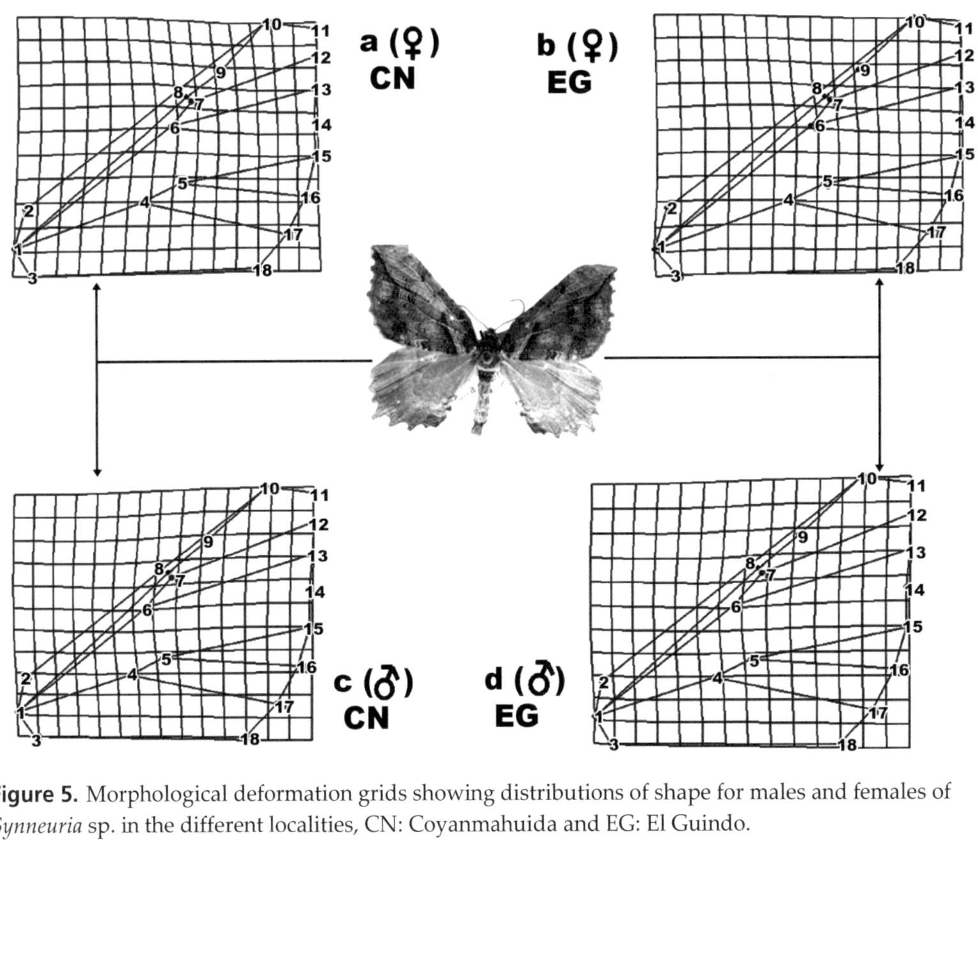

Figure 5. Morphological deformation grids showing distributions of shape for males and females of *Synneuria* sp. in the different localities, CN: Coyanmahuida and EG: El Guindo.

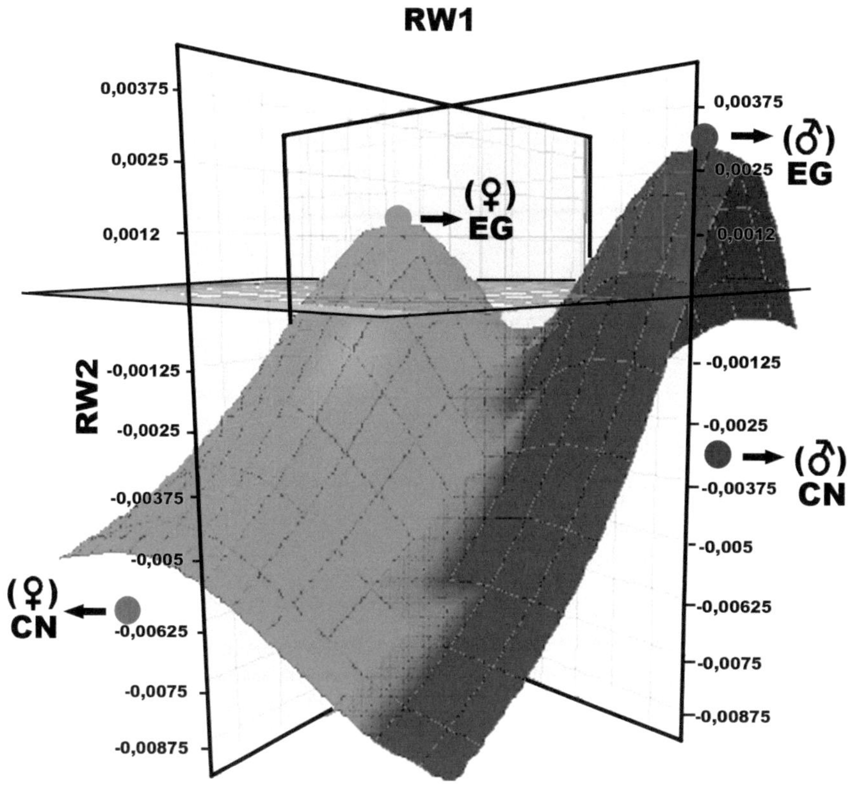

Figure 6. 3-D dispersion graph of shape variables by sex and locality in moths of the genus *Synneuria*. The points in the dark area indicate populations of males from El Guindo and Coyanmahuida, respectively, and in the clear area females from El Guindo and Coyanmahuida. ** Each point within the volumetric sector indicates a variable with different shape.

4.3. Discussion Case 1 and 2

The adoption of new techniques to determine variation in shape of both animals and plants is currently a widely discussed issue [69,70]. Geometric morphometrics can unify methodologies to quantify and visualize shape in all the ways that are possible.

For case 1, geometric morphometric was capable of detecting variation between species that are not clearly visible on plain sight, but rather at a sexual selection level between species. However, small variations on body shape could mark the difference in both populations, and these were proven according to Procustes distances and also by means of variance analyses. It is worth noting that the populations studied were subject to climate differences based on the different mountain ranges from which individuals were collected.

Although these differences are not obvious, individuals of the Coast Range had less thickened bodies than those of the Andes foothills. It has been reported that a climate with high relative humidity and constant temperatures promotes a thinner, subelytral cavity; this result was therefore expected for the Coast Range. The individuals of the Andes foothills had more visible morphological variations, which may be a consequence of the instability of the environment in this area (more variation in temperature, leading to thicker subelytral cavities). However, in spite of the climatic differences between populations there were not large morphological differences in the sexual dimorphism between populations. We may infer from this that gene flow has not been interrupted between them [17].

Regarding the case of Lepidoptera wing, it was very similar to the findings in beetles, but in this case differences were determined by means of small variations in wing shape associated with venation and flying styles of males and females [18].

For a number of authors, the variation in wing shape does not provide sufficient evidence to conclude that this is only a product of sexual dimorphism. It is frequently argued that individual variation in shape may be strongly dependent on environmental conditions [3,71]. However, our study showed a significant difference in wing shape between sexes, both within and between localities. Therefore, we conclude that the differences found here are analytical for the species and areas studied.

The differences among the individual configurations of each sex were captured using mathematical functions varying according to the position of each landmark in the wing image. These differences were located in landmarks 5, 6, 7 and 8, respectively. The geometric variation detected showed that the landmarks located on the base of the radial veins were key characters to distinguish different wing morphotypes among populations and sexes. The crucial attributes for the group would benefit the dispersion, migration and sexual selection; in males for the nuptial flight, territoriality and sexual selection, and in females primarily as a characteristic flight behaviour in the search for host plants e.g. [72-75]. Therefore, selection would act on wing shape to optimize flight characteristics [76].

5. Conclusions

This revision is intended to provide a wide view of GM use in some of the diverse study areas of sexual dimorphism in insects, confirming that by using the new tools that define shape as a differentiation characteristic it is possible to determine variations at minimum scales, which can be explained by means of sexual selection. Furthermore, by using geometric morphometric, besides identifying variations regarding sex, the researcher may determine relations between anatomic points of shape, in order to identify asymmetry patterns and generate hypotheses about the group development stability, [55,77]. Therefore, it is worth noting that in recent years research efforts have increased exponentially, and GM gains attention every day as a usefull tool for quantitative integration in morphology study due to its easy, inexpensive and fast application. Consequently, scientists are taking steps to combine these advanced techniques of morphometry study, to unify methodologies with molecular and genetic studies, in order to get results with total evidence within the analysis itself.

Author details

Hugo A. Benítez
Faculty of Life Sciences, University of Manchester, Manchester, UK
Instituto de Alta Investigación, Universidad de Tarapacá, Chile

Acknowledgement

To Dr. Viviane Jerez and Dr. Luis Parra of Zoology Department, Universidad de Concepción. Chile, for their comments and cooperation to generate the articles that were the core of the chapter and Ms. María Raquel Lazo de la Vega for her careful revision of the language.

6. References

[1] Adams C, Rohlf J, Slice D. Geometric morphometrics: ten years of progress following the "revolution". Italian Journal of Zoology 2004;71 5-16.
[2] Bookstein FL. A hundred years of morphometrics. Acta Zoologica Academiae Scientiarum Hungaricae 1998;44 7-59.
[3] Adams D, Funk DJ. Morphometric inferences on sibling species and sexual dimorphism in *Neochlamisus bebbianae* leaf beetles: Multivariate applications of the thin-plate spline. Systematic Biology 1997;46(1) 180-194.
[4] Dryden I, Mardia K. Statistical Shape Analysis. Chichester: Wiley; 1998.
[5] Kendall DG. The diffusion of shape. Advances in Applied Probability 1977;9 428-430.
[6] Bookstein F, Chernoff B, Elder R, Humphries J, Smith G, Strauss R. Morphometrics in evolutionary biology. Michigan: The Academy of Natural Sciences of Philadelphia; 1985.

[7] Zelditch ML, Swiderski D, Sheets D, Fink WL. Geometric Morphometrics for Biologists: A Primer. London: Elsevier; 2004.
[8] Rohlf FJ, Slice D. Extensions of the Procrustes method for the optimal superimposition of landmarks. Systematic Zoology 1990;39(1) 40-59.
[9] Rohlf FJ, Loy A, Corti M. Morphometric analysis of Old World Talpidae (Mammalia, Insectivora) using partial warp scores. Systematic Biology 1996;45(3) 344-362.
[10] Rohlf FJ. Shape statistics: Procrustes superimpositions and tangent spaces. Journal of Classification 1999;16 197-223.
[11] Gannon WL, Rácz GR. Character displacement and ecomorphological analysis of two long-eared *Myotis* (*M. auriculus* and *M. evotis*). Journal of Mammalogy 2006;87(1) 171-179.
[12] Koehl M. When does morphology matter?. Annual Review of Ecology and Systematics 1996;27 501-542.
[13] Cepeda-Pizarro J, Vega S, Vásquez H, Elgueta M.. Morfometría y dimorfismo sexual de *Elasmoderus wagenknechti* (Liebermann) (Orthoptera: Tristiridae) en dos eventos de irrupción poblacional. Revista Chilena de Historia Natural 2003;76 417-435.
[14] Andersson M. Sexual selection. Princeton: Princeton University Press; 1994.
[15] Moller AP, Zamora-Muñoz C. Antennal asymmetry and sexual selection in a cerambycid beetle. Animal Behaviors 1997;54 1509-1515.
[16] Cepeda-Pizarro JG, Vásquez H, Veas H, Colon GO. Relaciones entre tamaño corporal y biomasa en adultos de Tenebrionidae (Coleoptera) de la estepa costera del margen meridional del desierto chileno. Revista Chilena de Historia Natural 1996;69 67-76.
[17] Benítez H, Vidal M, Briones R, Jerez V. Sexual dimorphism and population morphological variation of *Ceroglossus chilensis* (Eschscholtz) (Coleoptera, Carabidae). Journal of the Entomological Research Society 2010a;12(2) 87-95.
[18] Benítez H, Briones R, Jerez V. Intra and Inter-population morphological variation of shape and size of Ceroglossus chilensis (Eschscholtz, 1829) in Chilean Patagonia. Journal of Insect Science 2011b;11 98 1-9.
[19] Benítez H, Parra LE, Sepulveda E, Sanzana MJ. Geometric perspectives of sexual dimorphism in the wing shape of Lepidoptera: the case of *Synneuria* sp. (Lepidoptera: Geometridae). Journal of the Entomological Research Society 2011a;13(1) 53-60.
[20] Rohlf FJ, Marcus LF. A revolution in morphometrics. Trends in Ecology & Evolution 1993;8 129-132.
[21] Klingenberg CP. Novelty and "homology-free" morphometrics: What's in a name?. Evolutionary Biology 2008;35 186–190.
[22] Bookstein FL. Landmark methods for forms without land-marks: localizing group differences in outline shape. Medical Image Analysis 1997;1 225-243.
[23] Younker JL, Ehrlich R. Fourier biometrics: harmonic amplitudes as multivariate shape descriptors. Systematic Zoology 1977;26 336-342.
[24] Ferson S, Rohlf FJ, Koehn RK. Measuring shape variation of two-dimensional outlines. Systematic Zoology 1985;34 59–68.
[25] Styner M, Oguz I, Xu S, Brechbuehler C, Pantazis D, Levitt JJ, Shenton ME, Gerig G. Framework for the statistical shape analysis of brain structures using SPHARM-PDM.

The Insight Journal. 2006, 1–20. http://hdl.handle.net/1926/215 (accessed 11 July 2006). (accessed 2 September 2012).
[26] McPeek MP, Shen L, Torrey JZ, Farid H. The tempo and mode of 3-dimensional morphological evolution in male reproductive structures. American Naturalist 2008; 171(5) E158–178.
[27] Macleod N, Rose KD. Inferring locomotor behaviour in Paleogene mammals via Eigenshape analysis. American Journal of Science 1993;293(A) 300–355.
[28] MacLeod N. Generalizing and extending the eigen-shape method of shape space visualization and analysis. Paleobiology 1999;25 107–138.
[29] Zelditch ML, Fink WL, Swiderski DL. Morphometrics, homology and phylogenetics: quantified characters as synapomorphies. Systematic Biology 1995;44 179–189.
[30] Goodall CR. Procrustes methods in the statistical analysis of shape. Journal of the Royal Statistical Society B 1991;53 285–339.
[31] Moczek A, Emlen D. Male horn dimorphism in the scarab beetle, *Onthophagus taurus*: do alternative reproductive tactics favour alternative phenotypes?. Animal Behaviour. 2000;59 459-466.
[32] Eberhard W. Rates of egg production by tropical spiders in the field. Biotropica 1979;11 292-300.
[33] Brock T, Guinness F, Albon S. Red Deer: Behavior and Ecology of Two Sexes. Chicago: University of Chicago Press ;1982.
[34] Emlen S. Reproductive sharing in different kinds of kin associations. American Naturalist 1996;148 756-763.
[35] Fincke O, Waage J, Koenig W. Natural and Sexual Selection Components of Odonate Mating Patterns. Cambridge: Cambridge University Press; 1997.
[36] Gidaszewski N, Baylac M, Klingenberg C. Evolution of sexual dimorphism of wing shape in the *Drosophila melanogaster* subgroup. BMC Evolutionary Biology 2009;9 110.
[37] O'Higgins P, Johnson D, Moore W, Flinn R. The variability of patterns of sexual dimorphism in the hominoid skull. Experientia 1990;46 670-672.
[38] Valenzuela N, Adams D, Bowden R, Gauger A. Geometric morphometric sex estimation for hatchling turtles: a powerful alternative for detecting subtle sexual shape dimorphism. Copeia 2004;4 735-742.
[39] Pretorius E. Using geometric morphometrics to investigate wing dimorphism in males and females of Hymenoptera – a case study based on the genus *Tachysphex* Kohl (Hymenoptera: Sphecidae: Larrinae). Australian Journal of Entomology 2005;44 113-121.
[40] Taylor A. Size and shape dimorphism in great ape mandibles and implications for fossil species recognition. American Journal of Physical Anthropology 2006;129 82-98.
[41] O'Higgins P, Dryden IL. Sexual dimorphism in hominoids: fur-ther studies of craniofacial shape differences in Pan, Gorilla and Pongo. Journal of Human Evolution 1993;24 183-205.
[42] O'Higgins P, Collard M. Sexual dimorphism and facial growth in papionin monkeys. Journal of Zoology 2002;257 255-272.

[43] Leigh SR. Cranial ontogeny of Papio baboons (Papio hamadr-yas). American Journal of Physical Anthropology 2006;130 71-84.

[44] Schaefer K, Mitteroecker P, Gunz P, Bernhard M, Bookstein FL. Craniofacial sexual dimorphism patterns and allometry among extant hominids. Annals of Anatomy 2004;186(5-6) 471-478.

[45] Butler MA, Losos JB. Multivariate sexualdimorphism, sexual selection, and adaptationin Greater Antillean Anolis lizards. Ecological Monographs 2002;72(4) 541-559.

[46] Butler MA, Sawyer SA, Losos JB. Sexual dimorphism and adap-tive radiation in Anolis lizards. Nature 2007;447 202-205.

[47] Malmgren JC, Thollesson M. Sexual size and shape dimorphism in two species of newts, Triturus cristatus and T. vulgaris (Caudata: Salamandridae). Journal of Zoology 1999;249 127-136.

[48] Bonduriansky R. Convergent evolution of sexual shape dimor-phism in Diptera. Journal of Morphology 2006;267 602-611.

[49] Atchley WR. Components of sexual dimorphism in Chi-ronomus larvae (Diptera: Chironomidae). American Naturalist 1971;105(945) 455-466.

[50] Benítez H, Jerez V, Briones R. Proporción sexual y morfometría para dos poblaciones de *Ceroglossus chilensis* (Eschscholtz, 1829) (Coleoptera: Carabidae) en la Región del Biobío, Chile. Revista Chilena de Entomología 2010b;35 61-70.

[51] Alibert P, Moureau B, Dommergues J, David B. Differentiation at a microgeographical scale within two species of ground beetle, *Carabus auronitens* and *C. nemoralis* (Coleoptera, Carabidae): a geometrical morphometric approach. Zoologica Scripta 2001;30 299-311.

[52] Rohlf F. TPSdig, v. 2.12. NY: State University at Stony Brook; 2008a.

[53] Klingenberg C. MORPHOJ: an integrated software package for geometric morphometrics. Molecular Ecology Resources 2011;11 353-357.

[54] Jiroux E. Le genre Ceroglossus, vol.14. Magellanes: Collection Systematique; 2006.

[55] Klingenberg C, Barluenga M, Meyer A. Shape analysis of symmetric structures: quantifying variation among individuals and asymmetry. Evolution 2002;56 1909–1920.

[56] Allen CE, Zwaan BJ, Brakefield PM. Evolution of Sexual Dimorphism in the Lepidoptera. Annual Review of Entomology 2011;56 445–464.

[57] Stillwell RC, Blanckenhorn WU, Teder T, DavidowitzG, Fox CW. Sex differences in phenotypic plasticity affect variation in sexual size dimorphism in insects: from physiology to evolution. Annual Review of Entomology 2010;55 227–245.

[58] Esperk T, Tammaru T. Determination of female-biased sexual size dimorphism in moths with a variable instar number: the role of additional instars. European Journal of Entomology 2006;103 575–586.

[59] Tammaru T, Esperk T, Ivanov V, Teder T. Proximate sources of sexual size dimorphismin insects: locating constraints on larval growth schedules. Evolutionary Ecology 2010;24 161–175.

[60] Berger D, Walters R, Gotthard K. What limits insect fecundity? Body size- and temperature-dependent egg maturation and oviposition in a butterfly. Functional Ecology 2008;22 523–29.
[61] Fischer K, Fiedler K. Sex-related differences in reaction norms in the butterflyLycaena tityrus (Lepidoptera: Lycaenidae). Oikos 2000;90 372–80.
[62] Wiklund C, Karlsson B, Leimar O. Sexual conflict and cooperation in butterfly reproduction: a comparative study of polyandry and female fitness. Proceedings of the Royal Society B: Biological Sciences 2001;268 1661–67.
[63] Reeve JP, Fairbairn DJ. Change in sexual size dimorphism as a correlated response to selection on fecundity. Heredity 1999;83 697–706.
[64] Mutanen M, Kaitala A. Genital variation in a dimorphic moth *Selenia tetralunaria* (Lepidoptera, Geometridae). Biological Journal of the Linnean Society 2006;87(2) 297-307.
[65] Meyer-Rochow VB, Lau T. Sexual dimorphism in the compound eye of the moth *Operophtera brumata* (Lepidoptera, Geometridae). Invertebrate Biology 2008;127(2) 201–216.
[66] Sihvonen P. Mating behaviour and copulation mechanisms in the genus *Scopula* (Geometridae: Sterrhinae). Nota Lepidopterologica 2008;30(2) 299–313.
[67] Forrest TG. Insect size tactics and developmental strategies. Oecologia 1987;73 178-184.
[68] Rohlf FJ. TPSUtil, v. 1.40. NY: State University at Stony Brook; 2008b.
[69] http://life.bio.sunysb.edu/morph/ (accessed 2 September 2012)
[70] Lawing AM, Polly PD. Geometric morphometrics: recent applications to the study of evolution and development. Journal of Zoology 2010;280 1–7.
[71] Klingenberg CP. Evolution and development of shape: integrating quantitative approaches. Nature Reviews Genetics 2010;11 623–635.
[72] Tatsuta H, Mizota K, Akimoto SI. Allometric patterns of heads and genitalia in the stag beetle *Lucanus maculifemoratus* (Coleoptera: Lucanidae). Annals of the Entomological Society of America 2001;94 462–466.
[73] Dudley R. The Biomechanics of Insect Flight: Shape, Function, Evolution. Princeton: Princeton University Press; 2000.
[74] Breuker C, Brakefield PM, Gibbs M. The associations between wing morphology and dispersal is sex-limited in the Glanville fritillary butterfly *Melitaea conxia* (Lepidoptera: Nymphalidae). European Journal of Entomology 2007;104 445–452.
[75] Dockx C. Directional and stabilizing selection on wing size and shape in migrant and resident monarch butterflies, *Danaus plexippus* (L.), in Cuba. Biological Journal of the Linnean Society 2007;92 605–616.
[76] Johansson F, Soderquist M, Bokma F. Insect wing shape evolution:independent effects of migratory and mate guarding flight on dragonfly wings. Biological Journal of Linnaean Society 2009;97 362–372.
[77] DeVries PJ, Penz CM, Hill RI. Vertical distribution, flight behaviour and evolution of wing morphology in *Morpho* butterflies. Journal of Animal Ecology 2010;79 1077–1085.

[78] Klingenberg CP, McIntyre GS. Geometric morphometrics of developmental instability: analyzing patterns of fluctuating asymmetry with Procrustes methods. Evolution 1998;52 1363–1375.

Chapter 4

The History of Sexual Dimorphism in Ostracoda (Arthropoda, Crustacea) Since the Palaeozoic

Hirokazu Ozawa

Additional information is available at the end of the chapter

http://dx.doi.org/10.5772/55329

1. Introduction

Studies of the origin and history of sex in organisms are important for elucidating life-history strategies and reproductive modes, and are an essential component of the study of evolutionary biology [1]. Sexual dimorphism (*i.e.*, morphological differences between males and females) and its relationship to reproductive modes in both living and extinct/fossil organisms is a key aspect of such studies [2] [3].

Ostracods (Arthropoda) are the only organisms useful for investigations of the long-term history of sexual dimorphism during the last ca. 500 million years since the early Palaeozoic, *i.e.*, Ordovician (ca. 490 Ma = 490 million years ago) [4]. Ostracods are a class of small crustaceans (Figures 1 and 2) of which the adult form is around 1.0 mm in length, that inhabit most aquatic areas; *e.g.*, marine, brackish, and freshwater conditions (Figure 3) [5] [6]. Most ostracods have the ability to reproduce sexually, except for a part of species capable of reproducing asexually (parthenogenesis). The most distinctive feature of ostracods is the calcareous carapace (Figures 1 and 2). Species with strongly calcified carapaces are relatively easily fossilised, and ostracods are abundant in sediments globally starting from the early Ordovician [7]. In contrast, the proteinaceous (= 'chitinous') soft body with appendages (Figure 2) is rarely fossilised due to a lack of mineralised parts, and as a result an ostracod fossil typically consists only of the hard carapace. However, this is sufficient for both recent and fossil specimens to be identified to the species level, based on various carapace morphological characteristics (Figures 1 and 2).

Similar to other crustaceans such as decapods, ostracods grow by moulting (ecdysis; Figure 4). For example, in one ostracod order, the Podocopida, there are usually eight moult stages between egg and adult, with the last moulting being the first sexually mature stage. Carapace and appendage sexual dimorphism can be recognised during the last adult stage (Figures 5 and 6), and to a lesser degree in late juvenile stages [8–10].

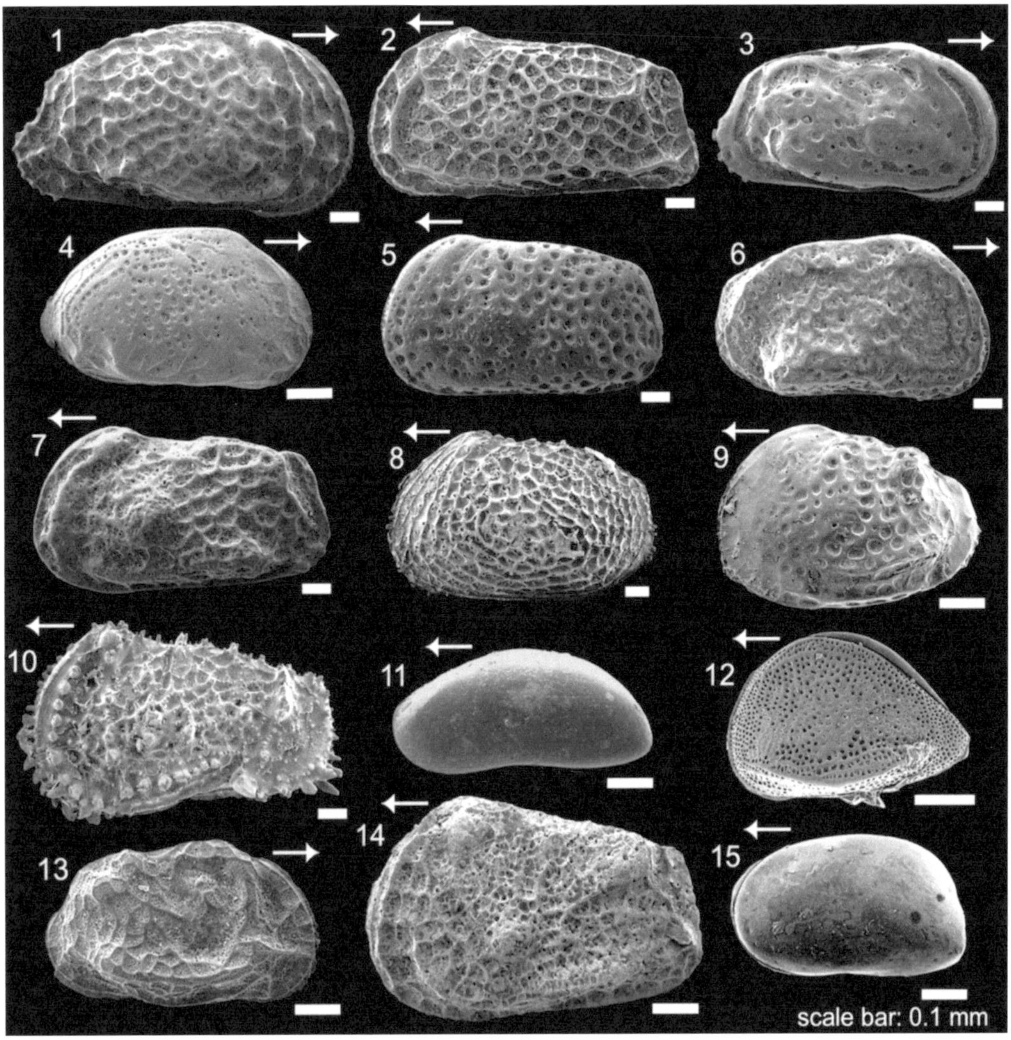

Figure 1. SEM images of fifteen ostracod species (Podocopida) from modern coast of southern Okhotsk Sea, modified from Ozawa (2012). 1: *Baffinicythere ishizakii*, RV, 2: *Baffinicythere robusticostata*, LV, 3: *Cornucoquimba alata*, RV, 4: *Howeina camptocytheroidea*, RV, 5: *Johnnealella nopporensis*, LV, 6: *Pectocythere* sp., RV, 7: *Laperousecythere robusta*, LV, 8: *Rabilimis septentrionalis*, LV, 9: *Robertsonites hanaii*, LV, 10: *Acanthocythereis dunelmensis* s.l., LV, 11: *Argilloecia toyamaensis*, LV, 12: *Cytheropteron carolae*, LV, 13: *Palmenella limicola*, RV, 14: *Elofsonella* cf. *concinna*, LV, 15: *Krithe* sp, LV. Arrows indicate anterior. LV: left valve, RV: right valve.

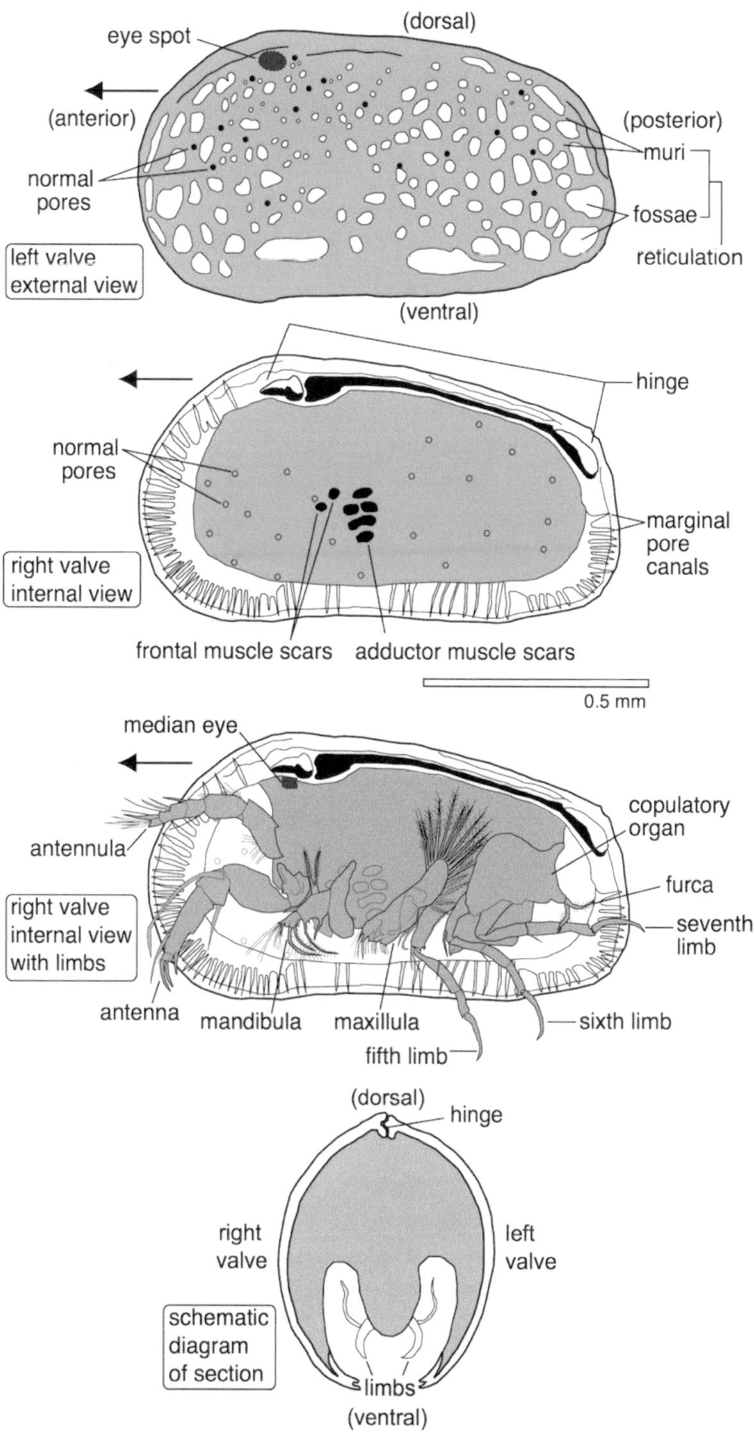

Figure 2. Morphology of ostracod male, based on *Hemicythere villosa* (Podocopida), modified from Horne *et al*. (2002)

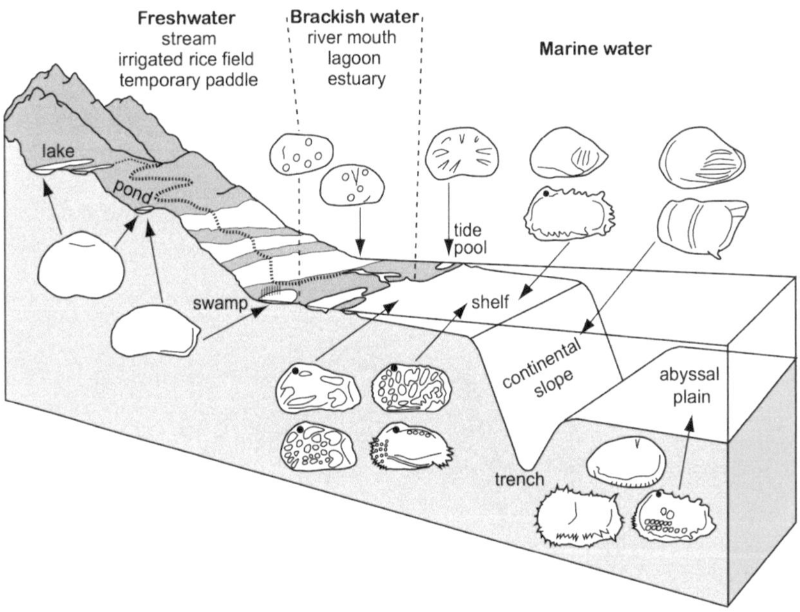

Figure 3. Schematic hypothetical profile of terrestrial aquatic to abyssal habitats of living ostracods progressing toward coastline, modified from Benson (2003).

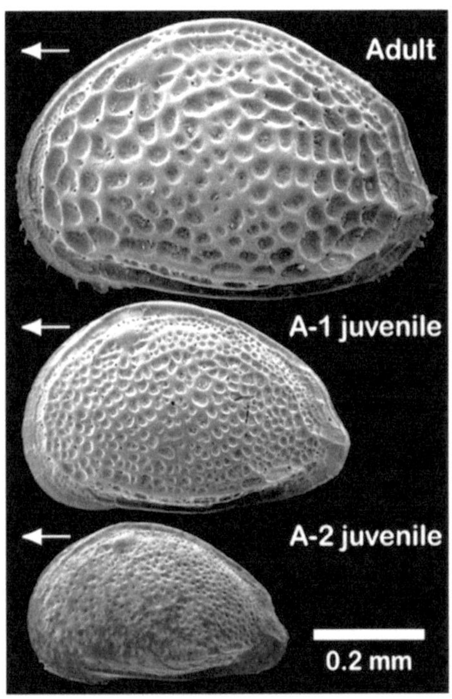

Figure 4. SEM images of last three molting stgaes in *Aurila* sp. of Ozawa and Kamiya (2009) (Podocopida) from the modern coast of northeastern Japan Sea, modified from Ozawa (2012). Arrows indicate anterior.

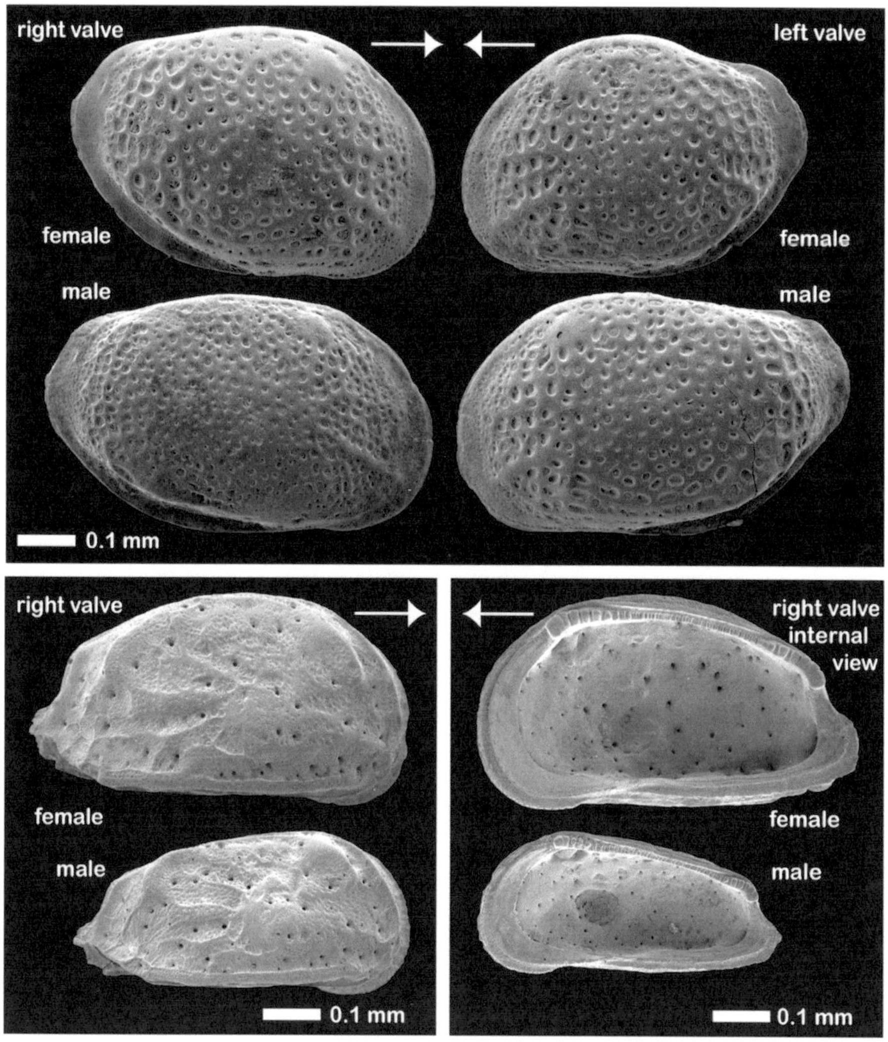

Figure 5. SEM images of carapaces in male and female of *Loxoconcha kamiyai* (upper two rows) and *Finmarchinella hanaii* (lower two rows) (Podocopida) from Quaternary deposits of central Japan, modified from Ozawa (2012). Arrows indicate anterior.

In organisms—other from ostracods—with abundant fossil records, there are very few cases of likely sexual dimorphism. One such case is the speculated "sexual dimorphism" of extinct ammonites (molluscs) discovered since the 1860s [11]. Many occurrences of ammonite fossils have been reported globally, and with respect to shell size, two different forms exist in particular groups of ammonites: the larger 'macroconch' and smaller 'microconch' within a probable single species from such genera as *Graphoceras, Ludwigina, Perisphinctes,* and *Yokoyamaceras* from Jurassic and Cretaceous strata [12–14].

However, ammonite sexual dimorphism has long been debated. In addition, whether microconchs of ammonites are males or females remains speculative [11] [15]; therefore, which ammonite form constitutes the male shell remains uncertain. In contrast, because ostracods are living organisms, we can examine their soft body and appendages in detail, including rarely fossilised parts such as the copulatory organs of males and females. Furthermore, we have excellent an fossil record of ostracods extending back to the early Palaeozoic, so we can compare modes of sexual dimorphism by comparing living to extinct fossil species. Therefore, we are able to determine the detailed characteristics associated with sexual dimorphism and their function in ostracods more easily than in extinct organisms such as ammonites.

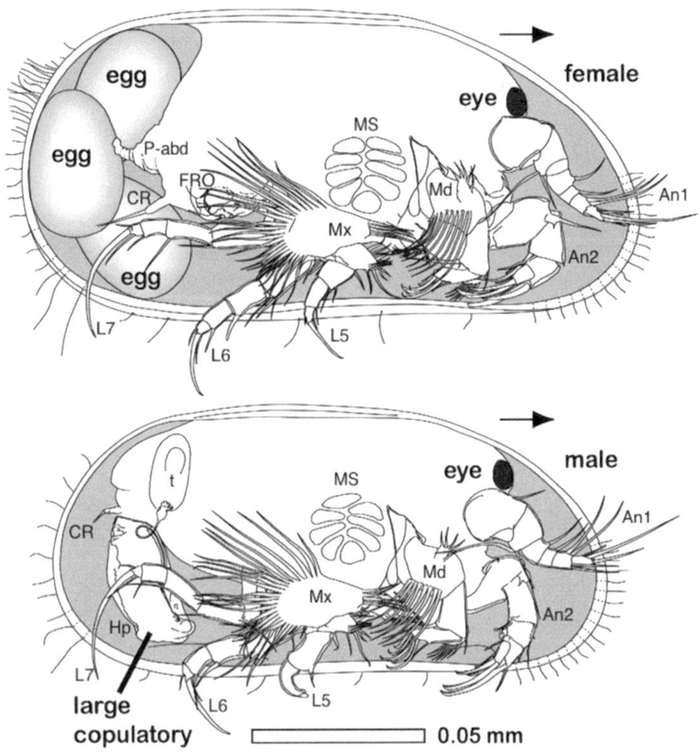

Figure 6. Morphology of female and male with right valve removed (one of each pair of appendages drawn for clarity) of *Vestalenula cornelia* (Podocopida) from modern springs in Yaku-shima Island of southwestern Japan, modified from Smith *et al.* (2006). Arrows indicate anterior.

Due to these unique traits, ostracods are the only organisms on earth that are useful for studying the history of sexual dimorphism since the Ordovician. Representative examples of sexual dimorphism within ostracods, mainly in species from Japan, are first introduced. This chapter then introduces one example of a sexually dimorphic feature accompanied by heterochrony (paedomorphosis). Recently, our research group found a rare case of sexual dimorphism in ostracod hingements with a paedomorphic character within only one phylogenetic group of one family. This morphology could be an important characteristic for evaluation of the history of sexual dimorphism in ostracods since the early Palaeozoic [16]. The author discusses this together with the history of ostracod sexual dimorphism from the

Palaeozoic to Recent, reviewing another case of ostracod sexual dimorphism with paedomorphosis reported by [17].

2. General features of ostracods for taxonomy, ecology, and morphology

Ostracods are a class of small crustaceans (Figures 1 and 2), the adult form of which is typically ca. 1.0 mm in length. They are not generally well known to many people except for researchers of fossils or living crustaceans due to their small size and lack of commercial significance compared to other crustaceans; *e.g.*, shrimps and crabs.

Class Ostracoda consists of the following six orders: Podocopida, Platycopida, Palaeocopida, Leperditicopida, Myodocopida, and Halocypridina [10]. This chapter focuses mainly on ostracod species belonging to the order Podocopida, which consists of more than 20,000 named living and fossil species distributed globally, because Podocopida is the most diversified taxonomic group in class Ostracoda (Figure 3) [10]. The well-known bioluminescent organism 'the sea firefly' (called 'umi-hotaru' in Japanese) is a kind of ostracod but belongs to another order, Myodocopida.

Ostracods occur in most aquatic environments on earth (Figure 3), such as the deep sea to a depth of several thousands of meters, through to shallow seas on the continental shelf [5]. They also live in rock pools in intertidal zones, brackish water areas at river mouths, lagoons and estuaries, freshwater lakes, ponds, irrigated rice fields, and temporary puddles. Most species are benthic throughout their lives, and crawl on or through the surface sediment and among aquatic plants [10]. A number of interstitial species, which live between sediment particles, are also distributed globally [18] [19].

The most distinctive feature of ostracods is the calcareous bivalved carapace (or shell), consisting of two valves that completely envelop the soft body and all appendages (Figures 1 and 2) [10]. Various types of appendage are protruded between opened valves for locomotion, feeding, and reproduction. The two valves (termed right and left) are connected by a hingement running along the dorsal margin (Figure 2). The word ostracod (or 'ostracode') is derived from Greek word 'ostrakon', which means 'a shell'. This carapace (or shell) has various morphological characteristics (Figures 1 and 2) that allow detailed taxonomic and phylogenetic studies to be performed on both living and fossil specimens [20–22].

Like other crustaceans such as decapods, ostracods grow by moulting (ecdysis; Figure 4). For example, in Podocopida, there are usually eight moult stages between egg and adult [20]. Species with strongly calcified carapaces, such as most marine species, are relatively easily fossilised. Ostracods are abundant in sediments globally, beginning in the early Ordovician (ca. 490 Ma) [7]. The proteinaceous (= 'chitinous') soft body and appendages are rarely fossilised due to a lack of mineralised parts, with rare exceptions, such as preservation of the soft parts of Silurian fossils [23]. Therefore, an ostracod fossil typically consists only of the hard-calcified carapace; however this is sufficient for identification of both modern and fossil specimens to the species level based on various carapace morphological characteristics.

In particular, the surface ornamentation (reticulation, fossae, muri, eye tubercle, ridges and so on), hingement type, muscle scar morphology (Figures 1 and 2), and pore shape and numbers are useful for ostracod taxonomy [24]. With living specimens, the morphology of male copulatory organs and other appendages are also used for species identification, similar to identification techniques used for other crustaceans, such as decapods [24–26]. Fossil ostracods are commonly utilised by palaeontologists as important palaeoenvironmental and stratigraphic (geological age) indices, and have long been used in oil and gas exploration [4] [27–29].

3. Representative examples of ostracod sexual dimorphism in extinct and living species

Like other crustaceans such as crabs, ostracods grow by moulting (ecdysis; Figure 4). For example, in Podocopida, there are usually eight moult stages between egg and adult, and the last moulting is the first sexually mature stage [20]. The adult stage is termed 'A', whereas juvenile stages are numbered; *e.g.*, 'A-1' (*i.e.*, one stage before the adult) and 'A-2' (two stages before the adult), as shown in Figure 4 [20]. Sexual dimorphism (morphological differences between males and females) is commonly found on carapaces and appendages [4, 9, 30], as shown in Figures 5 and 6, and is especially recognisable during the last adult stage (A), and to a lesser degree in the later juvenile stages, such as A-1.

This article introduces representative examples of sexual dimorphism in the last adult stage from the Palaeozoic to Recent, primarily in representative Podocopida from within and around Japan.

3.1. Carapace shape and size

3.1.1. Palaeozoic example in an extinct group

A well-known example of ostracod sexual dimorphism of the carapace exists in species of the family Beyrichiidae of the order Palaeocopida from the Ordovician to the Permian (Figure 7) [4] [31]. In many species of this family, distinct sexual dimorphism is seen in the adult stage; *i.e.*, females possess a large bulbous swelling in the antero-ventral part of each valve. These swellings that open internally into the domicilium found in species of this family are known as brood pouches (or cruminae) [25].

Species of this family were already extinct at the end of Palaeozoic, so various functions for this kind of pouch, including brood care, have been speculated [15]. Valves and carapaces of juvenile stages within this pouch were found in two species of the genus *Beyrichia* (*B. kloedini* and *B. jonesii*) in the family Beyrichiidae [25]. Based on the example of those two species, it became clear that these were probably brood pouches. An alternative (or perhaps double) function as buoyancy aids has been proposed by some researchers; thus firm evidence that all pouch types were used only for brood care has not yet been found [25]. It has been

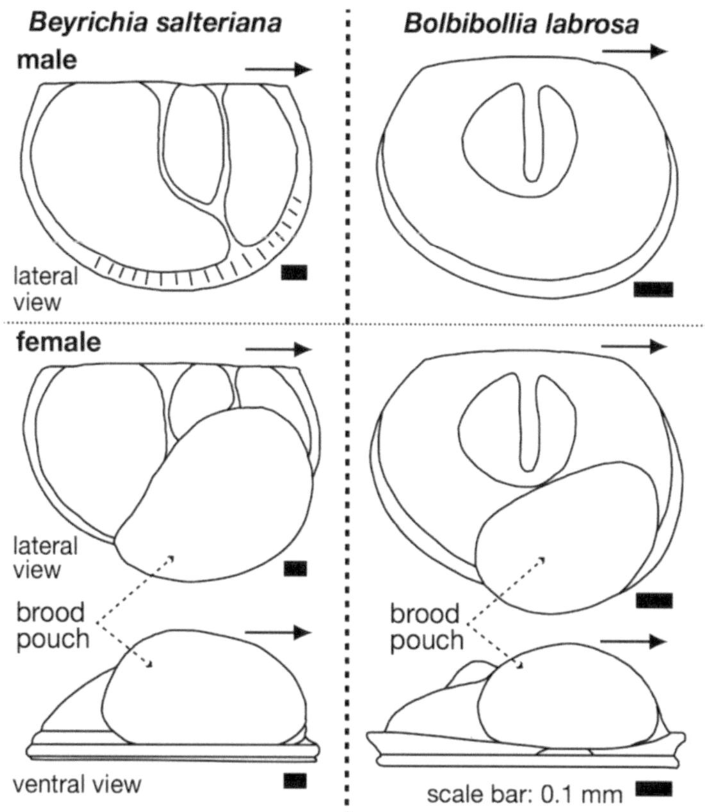

Figure 7. Carapace outlines of female and male of *Beyrichia salteriana* and *Bolbibollia labrosa* in Family Beyrichiidae (Palaeocopida) from Silurian deposits of Sweden and Canada respectively, modifed from Benson *et al.* (1961). Arrows indicate anterior.

inferred that species of this family inhabited Palaeozoic shallow-marine shelf-water environments [7]. Thus, a reasonable interpretation of pouch function in this family is needed to clarify the detailed evolutionary processes of the ecology and reproductive modes of Palaeocopida in Palaeozoic shallow-marine water areas.

3.1.2. Mesozoic example in an extinct species

Carapace shape and size sexual dimorphism is common in ostracods, and males can be larger or smaller than females [4]. One example from the Mesozoic is a non-marine species of the podocopid genus *Cypridea* [15] [32]. This genus occurred only during the Jurassic and Cretaceous, and is not found in Cenozoic deposits. The shape and size of *Cypridea subvaldensis* (Figure 8) from Cretaceous sediments in northeastern China was studied, and the differences between the two forms were recognised to represent sexual dimorphism within a single species [32].

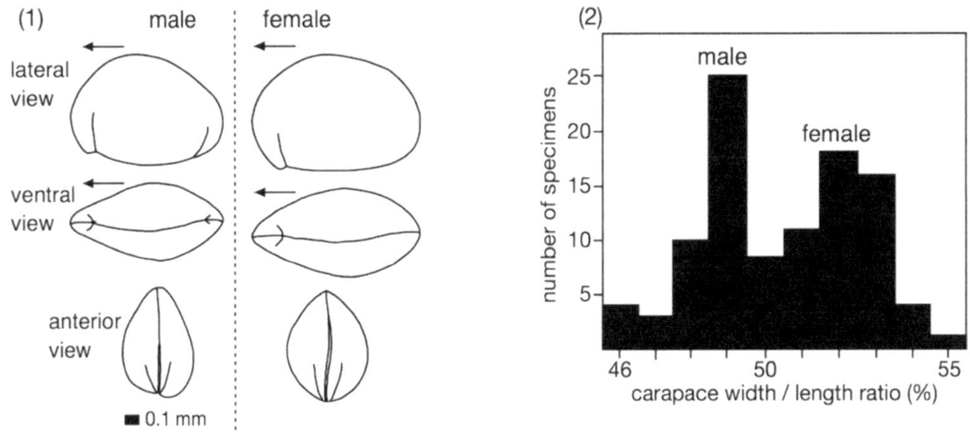

Figure 8. (1) Carapace outlines of female and male of *Cypridea subvaldensis* (Podocopida) in lateral, ventral and anterior views from Cretaceous deposits in northeastern China, modifed from Hanai (1951). Arrows indicate anterior. (2) Frequency of carapace length/ width ratio (%) for specimens of *Cypridea subvaldensis* in Cretaceous fossil assmblages from northeastern China, modifed from Hanai (1951).

Carapace sizes (length and width) of approximately 100 specimens of this species in one fossil assemblage from sedimentary rocks at one site were measured [32]. Based on the frequency of the carapace length/ width ratio, Hanai suggested that the two different-sized forms represent male and female forms within a single species. He proposed that the male carapace is smaller and narrower than that of the female, with a more arch-shaped outline along dorsal margin. This was based on the carapace shapes of the sexes of the single living species of a related genus, *Chlamydotheca,* in which the male form is slightly smaller and has a more arch-shaped dorsal margin than the female form.

3.1.3. Cenozoic and recent examples

A number of Japanese Cenozoic and living Podocopida genera, such as *Finmarchinella, Loxoconcha, Semicytherura* and *Vestalenula* (*e.g*., Figures 5 and 6), can be recognised by their distinct carapace shape and size sexual dimorphism [2, 9, 16, 17, 33]. In many cases, the male forms of these podocopids have relatively longer and narrower carapaces than the females (Figures 5 and 6) [34–36]. For example, in one modern species, *Bicornucythere bisanensis,* which is found in shallow brackish water areas in Japan, the male carapace is slightly more slender than that of the female (Figure 9) [8, 37, 38].

Primarily in podocopid species, female carapaces show greater posterior inflation than those of males, as in species of the genera *Metacypris* and *Xestoleberis* from Japan (Figure 10) [26] [39]. This kind of sexual dimorphism is more distinct in the adult than the juvenile stages [9]. In some cases, the male carapaces may be inflated posteriorly to accommodate relatively large copulatory organs, or it may have a more pronounced posterior keel, whereas in podocopid and myodocopid taxa with brood care, female carapaces are larger and more inflated than in the male [25] [40]. Eggs and the first two- or three-stage juveniles are retained within the posterior part of the domicilium. The shape of adult male valves of many Myodocopida species differ greatly from those of juveniles and females, and females are sometimes smaller than males even if there is brood care within the group [10].

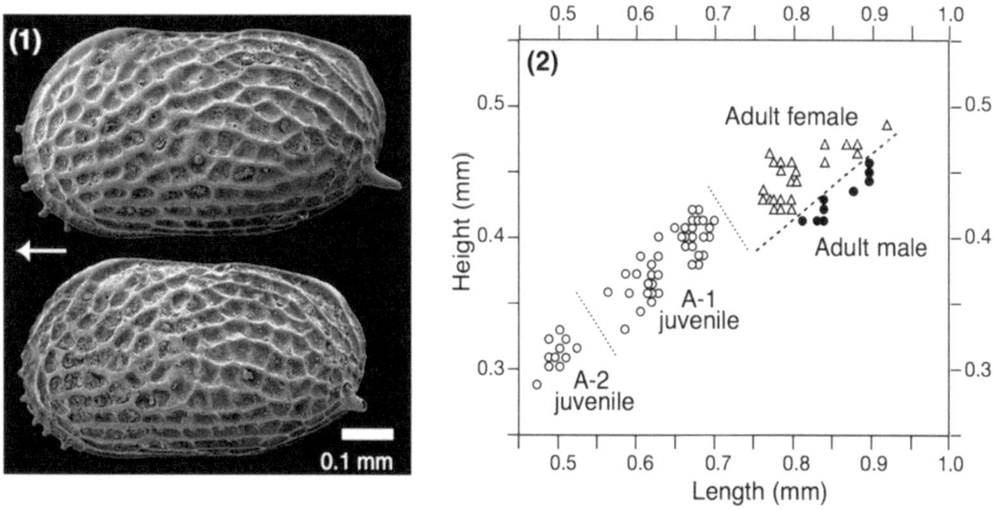

Figure 9. (1) SEM images of carapaces in male (upper) and female (lower) of *Bicornucythere bisanensis* (Podocopida) from Quaternary deposits of central Japan, modified from Ozawa (2009). Arrows indicate anterior. (2) Diagram for valve size (length and height) of this species in adult female, adult male, A-1 and A-2 juveniles, modified from Ozawa (2009).

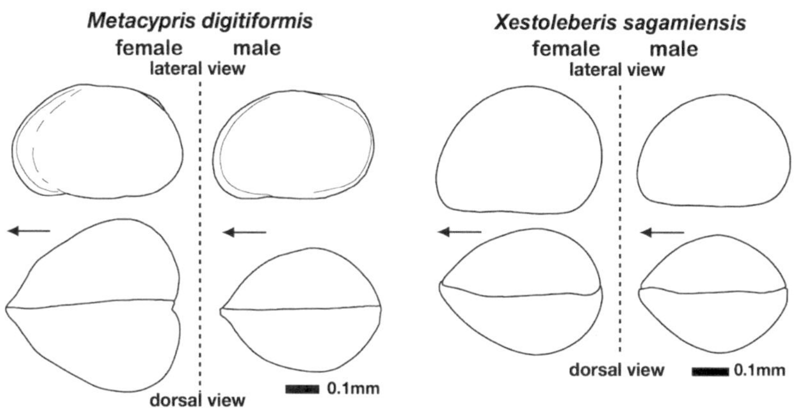

Figure 10. Carapace outlines of female and male in lateral and dorsal views of *Metacypris digitiformis* and *Xestoleberis sagamiensis* (Podocopida) from modern water areas of central Japan, redrawn from Smith and Hiruta (2004) and Sato and Kamiya (2007) respectively. Arrows indicate anterior.

The sexual behaviour of ostracods is diverse, and seven different types of brood care have been recognised in various lineages from Palaeozoic to Recent [25] [41]. These various types have arisen independently in several marine and non-marine lineages of ostracods, so diverse carapace shapes acting as brood pouches are found. The ability of the ostracod female to brood eggs or juveniles within the carapace might protect the young from severe environmental fluctuations and predation [25]. Brood care may be advantageous for the dispersal of some groups of non-marine water ostracods, such as species in the subfamily Timiriaseviinae (*e.g.*, genus *Metacypris*), the eggs of which may not be desiccation-resistant. The variety of brood care modes and carapace brood pouches that evolved in unrelated ostracod lineages is one of the most remarkable reproductive characteristics of ostracods, because other crustaceans exhibit a limited number of brood-care solutions [25] [42].

3.2. Carapace surface ornamentation

The podocopid species *Callistocythere pumila* favours very shallow brackish water environments around 1 m depth in inner bay and open lagoon areas near river mouths in Japan [43] [44]. It can be recognised by its conspicuous sexual dimorphism of carapace surface ornamentation (Figure 11). The female form has relatively distinct ornamentations on the entire carapace, such as numerous deep fossae [43] [44]. However, the male form has an extensive weakly ornamented area, especially in the median part of the carapace on a relatively slender valve (Figure 11).

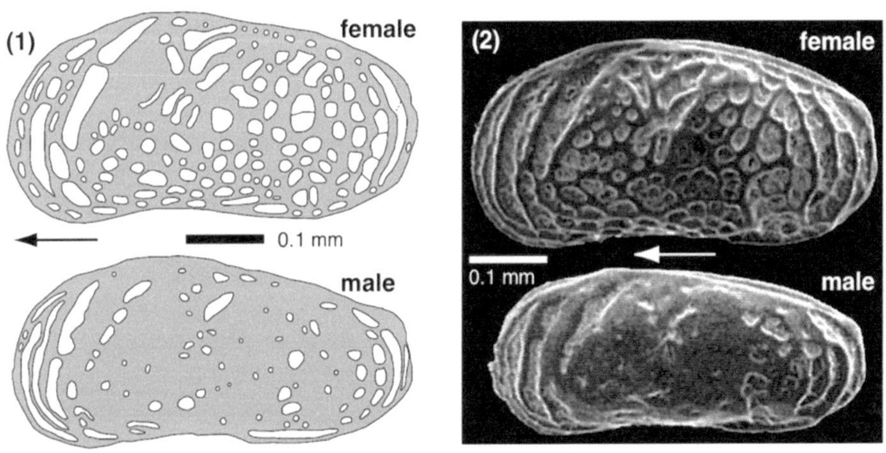

Figure 11. (1) Schematic patterns of fossae on carapace surface in female and male of *Callistocythere pumila* (Podocopida) in lateral view from modern brackish water area of central Japan, redrawn from Tsukagoshi (1998). (2) SEM images of carapaces in male and female of this species in lateral view, from modern brackish water area of central Japan, modified from Kamiya *et al.* (2001). Arrows indicate anterior.

The carapace morphology of this species occupies an intermediate taxonomic position between two genera, *Callistocythere* and *Leptocythere*; the female and male forms resemble the former and latter genera, respectively [43]. Due to these morphological differences between males and females, they were originally described as a different species [45] [46]. However, those two forms have recently been considered to represent males and females of a single species, *Callistocythere pumila*, based on the detailed description of soft parts [43]. As yet no reasonable interpretation of the function of sexually dimorphic ornamentation has been postulated. The significance of this dimorphism for the ecology or life-history of *C. pumila* requires investigation to clarify the detailed evolutionary processes of the ecology of Cenozoic brackish water podocopids.

3.3. Appendages

3.3.1. *The example of Bicornucythere bisanensis*

Bicornucythere bisanensis (Podocopida) predominantly inhabits shallow brackish water areas in inner bay areas near river mouths in and around Japan [47]. Sexual dimorphism of the appendages of this species has been known since the 1910s [45, 48, 49]. The right fifth limb (= first thoracic leg) of the male is uniquely thicker and slightly shorter than the left fifth limb [30] [50]. The central podomere of the right fifth limb is very inflated, and is 1.5-times the thickness of that of the female. Thus, the fifth limb of the male in this species shows asymmetry, and this unique morphology has not been observed in the female. This is a representative example of sexual dimorphism in podocopid appendages.

The ecological function of this dimorphism has been clarified by [30] [50]. They observed its mating behaviour under experimental conditions from detailed video recordings. According to their observations (Figure 12), this short and thick podomere in the right fifth limb of the male is an adaptation for courting behaviour, where the male rotates the female's carapace three or four times using the right fifth limb just before mating (Figure 12). Thus, this right limb (especially the central podomere) is thicker and shorter than both the male left limb and the female's fifth limb to facilitate holding and rotating the female carapace. The thick podomere of the male right fifth limb is markedly more muscular than either that of the left side and those of the female, facilitating this behaviour [15, 30, 37].

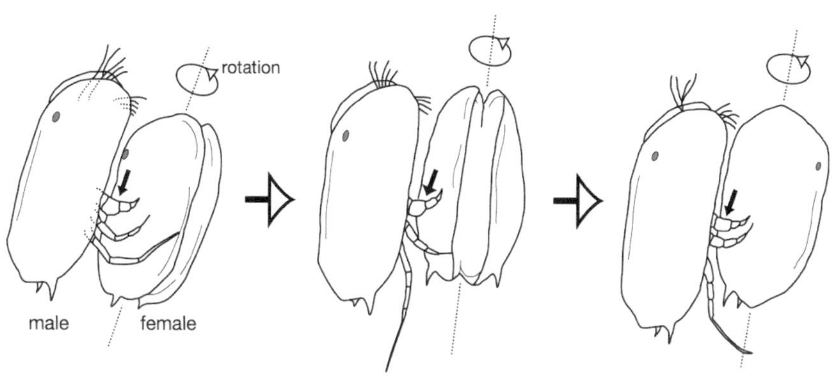

Figure 12. Schematic profile of courting behaviour (= rotation of female carapace by male's fifth limb) just before mating behaviour, indicating the location of its fifth limb by black arrows, for modern *Bicornucythere bisanensis* (Podocopida) from modern inner bay area of central Japan, modified from Abe and Vannier (1991).

3.3.2. *The example of Vargula hilgendorfi*

Several examples of sexual dimorphism of appendages other than the fifth limb in living marine species have been reported for *Vargula hilgendorfi* (Myodocopida) [51]. This species inhabits shallow marine water environments, and the relative size of the furca at the posterior part of the soft body compared to the length of the entire carapace differs between the sexes. The male's furca is relatively larger than that of the female. According to detailed observations of its ecological behaviour under experimental conditions [51], this species pushes off from sea-bottom sediments just before swimming in water, especially using the furca (Figure 13). Based on observations of video recordings, the male tends to swim around much more actively than the female; thus explaining the function of the relatively large furca in the male [37].

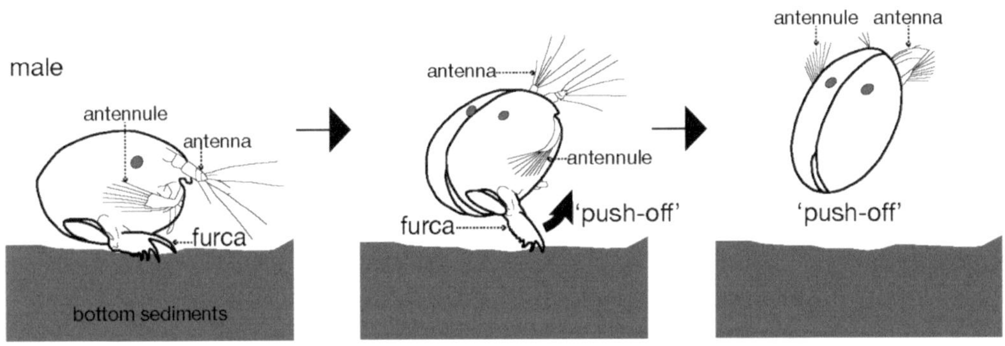

Figure 13. Schematic profile of 'push-off' behaviour just before swimming for modern *Vargula hilgendorfi* (Myodocopida), indicating the location of its furca by black arrows, modified from Vannier and Abe (1993).

A further four examples of sexually dimorphic appendages and eyes are found on *Vargula hilgendorfi*, as follows: (a) the existence or absence of two suckers on the first appendage (antennule), (b) different numbers of bristles on the first appendage, (c) different sizes of the basal part of the second appendage (antenna), (d) different sizes of compound eyes [37, 51]. The probable function of (a) is support by the male form of the female carapace during mating behaviour. However, the functions of the other sexually dimorphic characteristics (b)–(d) remain unclear. The Myodocopida first appeared during the early Palaeozoic (Ordovician), and still inhabit many marine environments [7]. Therefore, these other sexually dimorphic characteristics are interesting examples of myodocopid ostracod morphology, and indicate the evolutionary processes associated with their ecology, including mating behaviour and reproduction modes, since the Palaeozoic.

4. Sexual dimorphism in the inner carapace, with Paedomorphosis

Sexually dimorphic and paedomorphic morphological characteristics of the inner carapace were recently reported in two unrelated podocopid taxonomic groups from Japan [16] [17]. These, together with their ecological and evolutionary significance for ostracods since the Palaeozoic, are reviewed below.

4.1. Hingement morphology and dimorphism

The genus *Loxocorniculum* of the family Loxoconchidae was established [65] based primarily on modern *Loxocorniculum fischeri* from the Caribbean Sea, and is characterised by a horn-like protuberance on the postero-dorsal corner of the carapace. However, except for the horn-like protuberance, the carapace appearance of species of this genus, including *Loxocorniculum mutsuense* from Japan, is very similar to that of the genus *Loxoconcha* as noted by Ishii *et al.* [63]. The phylogenetic independence of *Loxocorniculum* in Japan as a genus distinct from *Loxoconcha* has been debated [16]. Therefore this chapter tentatively includes *Loxocorniculum mutsuense*, first proposed as a new species from Japan by [66], in the genus *Loxoconcha* following the opinion of Ishii *et al.* [63].

The ostracod genus *Loxoconcha* (family Loxoconchidae) is widely distributed in shallow marine environments from tropical to subarctic regions [52–54]. This is one of the most diversified ostracod genera, which comprises ca. 600 species [7]. This genus is common in and around Japan [55–59], and about 40 living and fossil species have been described [60]. Thus, *Loxoconcha* is one of the most important Japanese ostracod genera.

A new fossil species *Loxoconcha kamiyai* from Pleistocene strata from the eastern coast of the Sea of Japan (Figure 14) was described, and its carapace morphology examined [16]. Palaeobiogeography of *L. kamiyai* was discussed, and its phylogenetic relationship to related

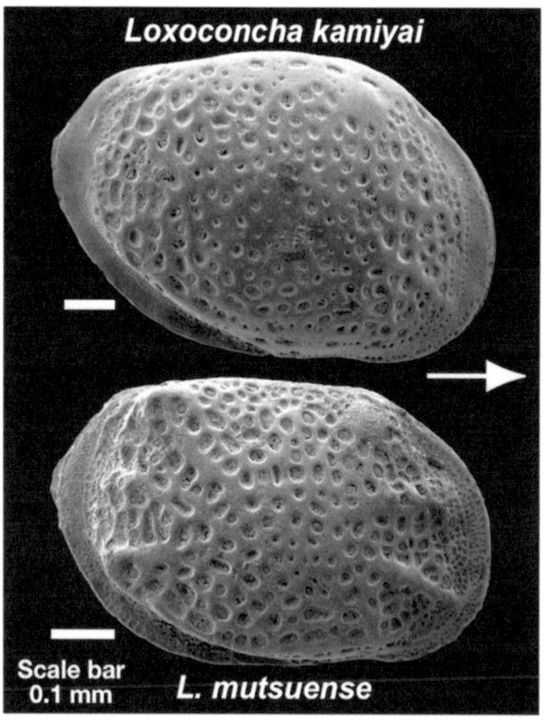

Figure 14. SEM images of two *Loxoconcha* species (Podocopida) from Quaternary deposits of central Japan, modified from Ozawa (2010). Arrows indicate anterior.

loxoconchid species was assessed, based on the pore distribution pattern (a type of ostracod sensory organ; Figure 15). The number, distribution, and differentiation of pores on the ostracod carapace surface during ontogeny have been studied to determine phylogenetic relationships among species [61]. The reconstruction of ostracod phylogeny based on pore analyses was first proposed by [21] for 14 species of the genus *Cythere*. His work was followed by [26] [62–64] for species of other genera. This method of phylogenetic reconstruction, proposed by [21], was termed 'differentiation of distributional pattern of pore (DDP) analysis' [61]. The pore distribution in *L. kamiyai* was examined by this method [16], and the results were compared to the pore data of 17 other *Loxoconcha* species (Figure 16).

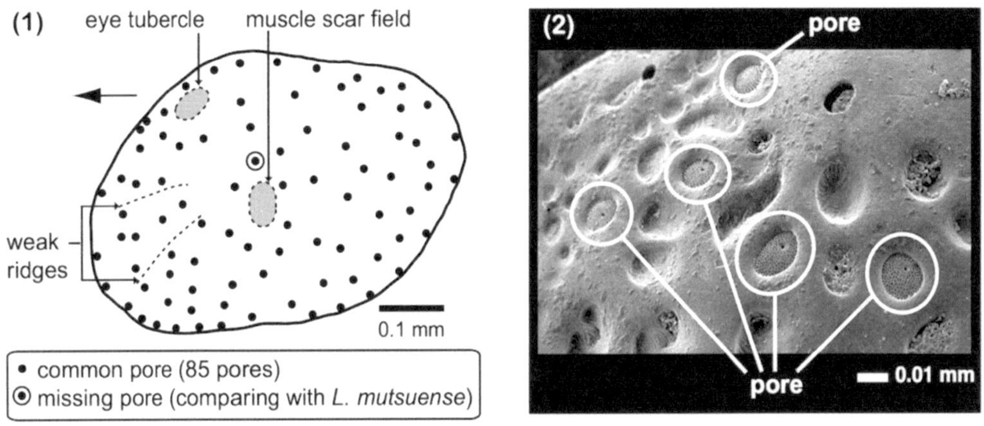

Figure 15. (1) Distribution pattern of pores in adult left valve of *Loxoconcha kamiyai* (Podocopida), modified from Ozawa and Ishii (2008). Position of one missing pore of this species is determined by comparison with the distribution pattern of pores of *Loxoconcha mutsuense* (= *Loxocorniculum mutsuense*; Podocopida) in Ishii *et al.* (2005). Arrows indicate anterior. (2) Close-up view of SEM images of pores in antero-dorsal marginal area on left valve of *Loxoconcha kamiyai* (Podocopida) from Quaternary deposits of central Japan, modified from Ozawa (2010).

On the basis of the DDP results for its adult and A-1 juvenile stages, *L. kamiyai* was determined to be the species most closely related to *Loxoconcha mutsuense* (= *Loxocorniculum mutsuense*). Both species have the same total number of pores on the carapace at the A-1 juvenile stage (75 pores per valve; Figure 16). The difference in total number of pores in the adult stage is only one between these two species, missing on the central area in *L. kamiyai* (Figure 15). These results strongly suggest its closest phylogenetic affinity to another species, *L. mutsuense,* in the same family [16].

Both *Loxoconcha kamiyai* and *Loxoconcha mutsuense* show a unique and remarkable sexual dimorphism in the adult stage, especially in the anterior element of the hingement (Figures 17 and 18). On the right valve, the anterior hingement element of the adult male is commonly smaller and rounder than that of the adult female. Its shape is very similar to the small, round anterior element of its A-1 juvenile stage [16]. The anterior element of the female hingement is larger and more rectangular than that of either the male or the A-1 juvenile (Figures 17 and 18).

These morphological characteristics of *Loxoconcha kamiyai* are seen in specimens from diverse geological ages and geographical regions (Figure 19); in fossil specimens from Pliocene sediments (4–3 Ma) in the Nagano and Niigata Prefectures of central Japan (age from [67–69]) and Pleistocene strata around 1.5 and 0.9 Ma from the Noto Peninsula and

Sado Island in central Japan (age from [70] [71]). The same hingement character is found in *L. mutsuense* of various geological ages in fossil specimens from many areas (Figure 20), such as Pleistocene strata around 1.5 and 0.9 Ma in central Japan [16], and also in modern specimens from shallow marine environments off the northeastern and southwestern Japanese coast [66] [72].

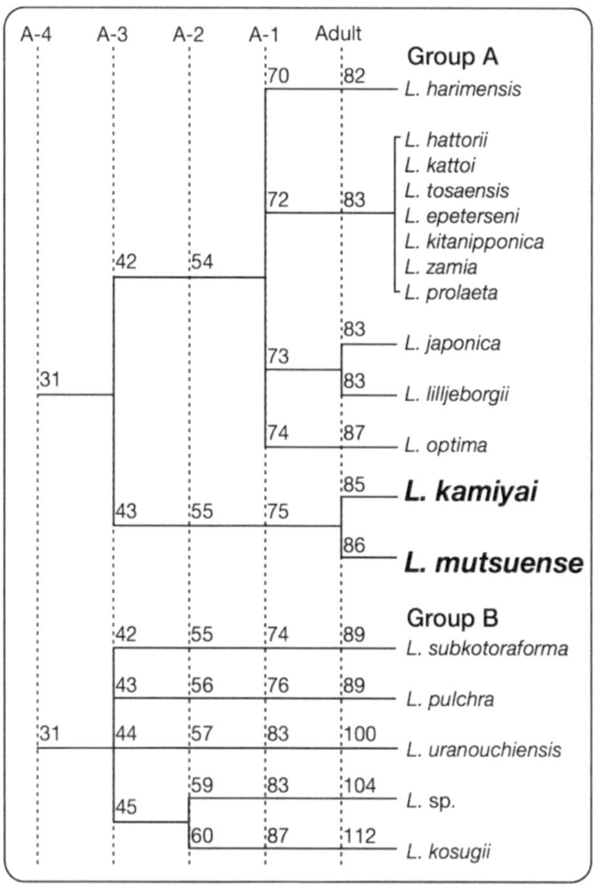

Figure 16. Results of DDP analysis for eighteen *Loxoconcha* species (Podocopida), modified from Ishii *et al.* (2005) and Ozawa and Ishii (2008). Numbers indicate total numbers of pores for each lineage and stage. Trees drawn by hand.

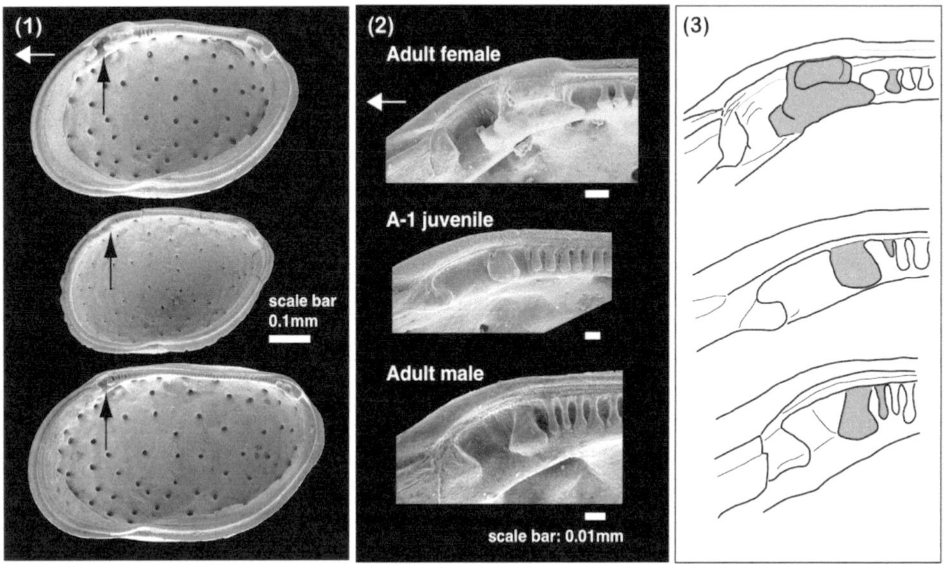

Figure 17. Comparison of lateral view (adult female, A-1 juvenile, adult male) of inner right valve of *Loxoconcha kamiyai* (Podocopida) from Quaternary deposits of central Japan, modified from Ozawa and Ishii (2008). (1): SEM images of lateral view from inside; arrows indicate locations of anterior hingement element, (2): SEM images of close-up view of anterior hingement element, (3): Sketch of anterior hingement element (= 2). Upper row: adult female, middle row: A-1 juvenile, lower row: adult male. White arrows indicate anterior.

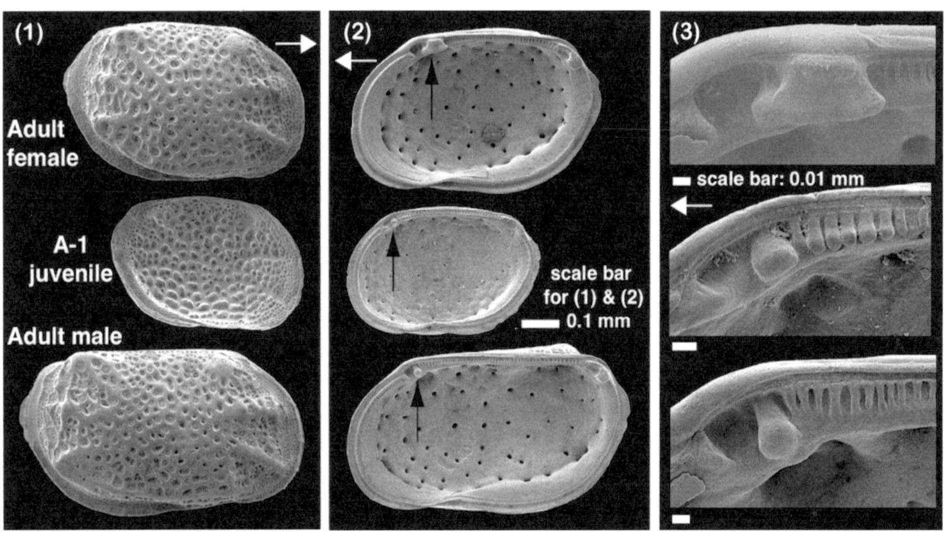

Figure 18. Comparison of SEM images of lateral view (adult female, A-1 juvenile, adult male) for right valve of *Loxoconcha mutsuense* (= *Loxocorniculum mutsuense*; Podocopida) from Quaternary deposits of central Japan, modified from Ozawa and Ishii (2008). (1): External lateral view, (2): Internal lateral view; arrows indicate locations of anterior hingement element, (3): Close-up view of anterior hingement element. Upper row: adult female, middle row: A-1 juvenile, lower row: adult male. White arrows indicate anterior.

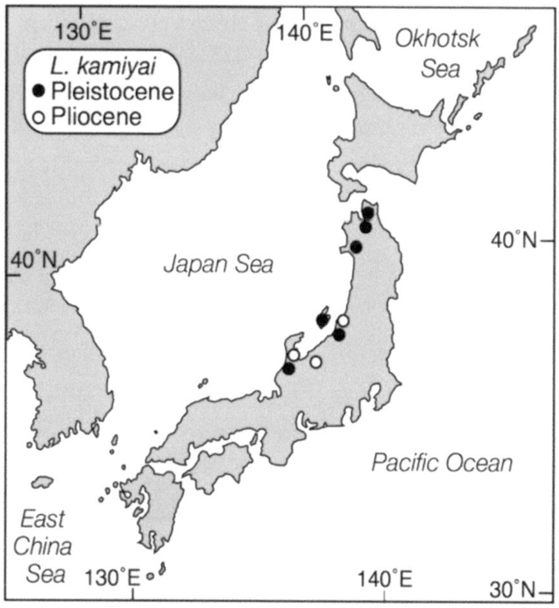

Figure 19. Geographical and geological occurrences of *Loxoconcha kamiyai* (Podocopida) based on data from previous studies, modified from Ozawa (2010).

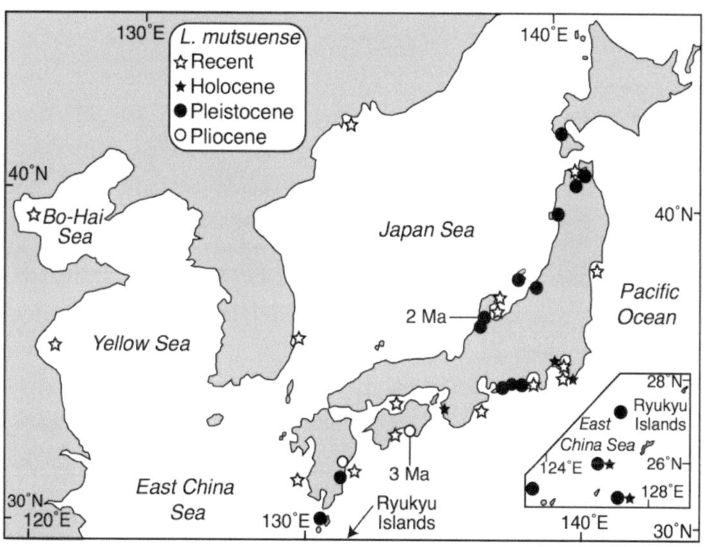

Figure 20. Geographical and geological occurrences of *Loxoconcha mutsuense* (= *Loxocorniculum mutsuense*; Podocopida) based on data from previous studies, modified from Ozawa (2010), adding with distributional data from southwestern Japan of Irizuki (2004).

This hingement sexual dimorphism in modern specimens of *Loxoconcha mutsuense* (= *Loxocorniculum mutsuense*) from the coast of northeastern Japan was mentioned only briefly in [66]. Ishizaki referred to a "hinge structure delicate in male but stronger (bold) in female with prominent tooth within anterior socket of right valve" ([66], p. 90) in the systematic description of this species. However, he did not show clear illustrations of these dimorphic characteristics for comparison. *L. mutsuense* from the coast of southwestern Japan was re-described in a carapace sketch from an internal view of the female right valve [72]. Okubo's illustration (Fig. 17b in [72], p. 425) clearly shows the large anterior hingement tooth on the female. However, he also did not refer to this characteristic or the morphology of the male's hingement in the text. Considering the findings of [16], Ozawa and Ishii concluded that this sexually dimorphic morphology is a stable characteristic within each species, and not a geographical or geological variation or a deformity within a single species.

Using the female's hingement as a standard, the male morphology in these two species can be explained as a type of heterochrony of [73] [74]; *i.e.*, paedomorphosis [16]. Paedomorphic examples of podocopid hingements have been found in two species in 11 pairs from five families—the Cytheridae, Leptocytheridae, Hemicytheridae, Cytheruridae, and Loxoconchidae—within the superfamily Cytheridea from the Miocene to the present [19, 75, 76]. This remarkable morphological difference in the anterior hingement element, between the sexes and the A-1 juvenile stage within the same species from one family, was first reported by [16].

This is likely why few publications include clear illustrations of ostracod hingements of male and female forms together with the A-1 juvenile stage, especially for ostracod taxa with a complex, rather than simple, hingement morphology; *e.g.*, adont and lophodont hingement types. We know of only one example of a detailed comparison of the number of teeth per gongylodont hingement in adult male and female forms with the A-1 juvenile of *Loxoconcha uranouchiensis* [9]. Further examples of the sexual dimorphism and paedomorphosis of the complicated hingement type will likely be found in other species or families of podocopid ostracods if hingements of male, female, and A-1 juveniles are precisely examined using SEM.

With regard to copulatory behaviour in *Loxoconcha kamiyai* and *L. mutsuense*, hingement sexual dimorphism does not appear to be directly related to functional morphology [16]. The anterior hingement element is located on the inner area of the carapace at the anterodorsal margin. This is farthest from the copulatory organ, which stretches out from the postero-ventral area between the two valves during mating (Figure 21) [16] [77]. Therefore, as yet there are no reasonable interpretations of the actual function of this kind of sexually dimorphic morphology.

Therefore, the mating and reproductive behaviours of the living species *Loxoconcha mutsuense* must be observed in detail by video recording, because the other species, *L. kamiyai*, has been extinct since the middle Pleistocene [16]. Such detailed observations will for the first time allow clarification of the actual function and significance of this dimorphism in their life-history. The significance for this dimorphism in the life-history or mating behaviour of the two species will facilitate elucidation of the evolutionary processes of the ecology and reproductive modes of shallow marine podocopids during the Cenozoic.

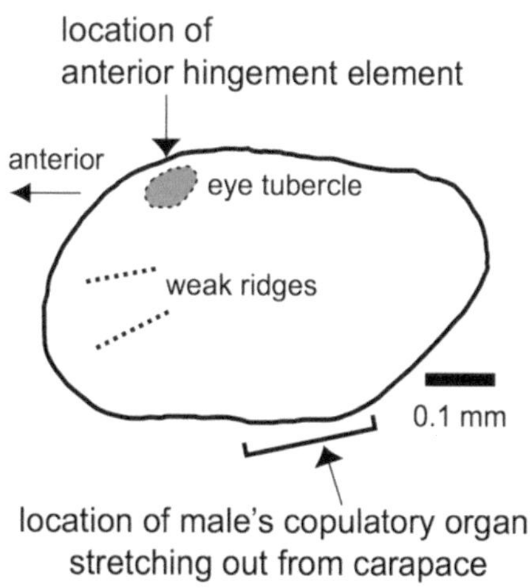

Figure 21. Schematic profile for location of anterior hingement element and inferred location of copulatory oragn stretching out from inner carapace for *Loxoconcha kamiyai* and *Loxoconcha mutsuense* (= *Loxocorniculum mutsuense*; Podocopida) in lateral view for left valve of male, based on observations for mating behaviour of other living *Loxoconcha* species (*L. japonica* and *L. uranouchiensis*) in Kamiya (1988b).

4.2. Example of the inner carapace with implications for the historical origin of the ostracod male

A type of sexual dimorphism with paedomorphosis in the inner marginal area of ostracod carapaces has been reported in the freshwater podocopid *Vestalenula cornelia*, of the family Darwinulidae [17], although this dimorphism was not found on the hingement (Figures 6 and 22). According to [17], the sexual dimorphism in *V. cornelia* is found along the ventral edge of the valve (Figure 22). The male has two internal tooth-shaped structures on the left valve, whereas the female has a single internal tooth on the left valve. Furthermore, the female has a keel-shaped structure on the right valve, which is absent from the male form (Figure 22). It is interesting that the A-1 juvenile has a similar arrangement to that of the adult male, in terms of carapace length–height and lateral outline [17]. Therefore, the male form of this species also exhibits paedomorphic morphology.

A speculative hypothesis to explain this interesting observation of paedomorphosis was proposed by [16], who suggested that the adult male forms of marine podocopid ostracods may have originated from adult female forms by paedomorphosis in ancient times; *i.e.*, the early Palaeozoic. The gongylodont hingement, characteristic of the family Loxoconchidae, is generally considered to be one of the most complex-shaped and derived hingements among all podocopid ostracod families since the late Cretaceous [7] [52]. Thus, the most derived hingement in loxoconchid ostracods would have by chance exhibited atavistic features. These may have been common in ancient and primitive ancestors of marine ostracods, although most podocopid species had already lost these characteristics by the early Cenozoic. Identification of this kind of sexual dimorphism in more complicated hingement shapes may be easier than in simpler and more primitive hingements, such as the adont or lophodont types.

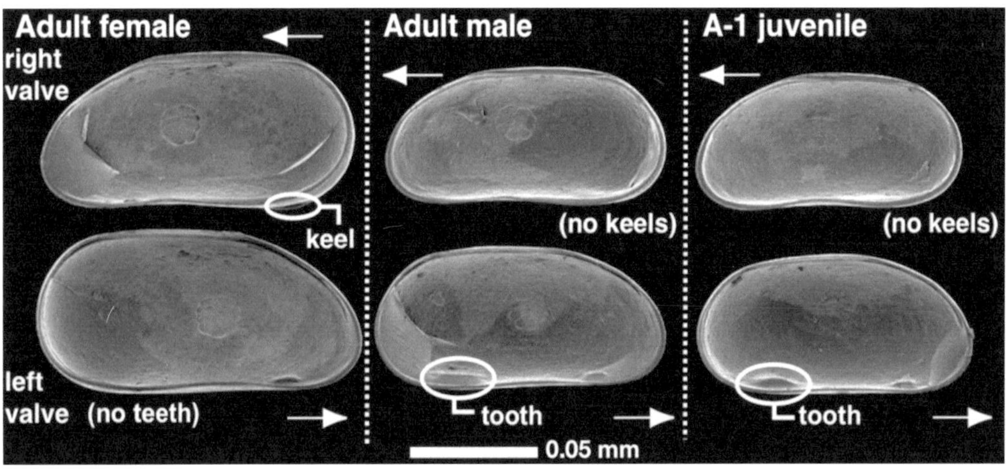

Figure 22. Comparison of SEM images of internal lateral view (adult female, adult male, A-1 juvenile) for right and left valves of *Vestalenula cornelia* (Podocopida) from modern springs in Yaku-shima Island of southwestern Japan, modified from Smith *et al.* (2006). Left column: adult female, central column: adult male, right column: A-1 juvenile, upper row: right valve, lower row: left valve. Arrows indicate anterior.

Non-marine ostracods are considered to have originated and diversified from marine ostracods multiple times, mainly during the Palaeozoic and Mesozoic [7]. Therefore, sexual dimorphism with paedomorphosis in the hingement of a marine species (*Loxoconcha kamiyai*) and in structures on the internal ventral margin of a freshwater species (*Vestalenula cornelia*) may provide insight into the origin of the ostracod male and the post-Palaeozoic history of ostracod sexual dimorphism with paedomorphosis [16]. Therefore, more data regarding the sexually dimorphic characteristics of ostracod carapaces (or appendages as much as possible) of many taxonomic groups, accompanied by heterochronic morphology since the early Palaeozoic, should be collected. Additionally, the excellent marine and non-marine ostracod fossil records since the Ordovician that are extant worldwide should be further researched.

5. Summary and future work

1. Many ostracod species have the ability to reproduce sexually, and are relatively easily fossilised because due to their highly calcified carapaces. Ostracods are abundant in sediments ranging from the Palaeozoic Ordovician (since ca. 490 million years ago) to the Cenozoic Holocene, in modern deposits. Considering these unique characteristics, ostracods represent useful tools for investigation of the history of sexual dimorphism of organisms on earth since the Ordovician. Many examples of ostracod sexual dimorphism, in terms of both shape and size, are evident on carapaces and appendages from the Palaeozoic to Recent.
2. Two podocopid species of the family Loxoconchidae (*e.g.*, *Loxoconch kamiyai*) show a unique sexual dimorphism in the adult stage on the anterior hingement element. Pore distribution patterns on their carapaces strongly suggest close phylogenetic affinities for these two species. Taking the female hingement morphology as a standard, male hingement can be explained in terms of a type of heterochrony; *i.e.*, paedomorphosis. Sexual dimorphism on the hingement accompanied by paedomorphosis occurs in only one phylogenetic group in this family, which is distinguished by the ontogenetic pore pattern distribution. This unique morphological feature may represent relict primitive characteristics of ancient ostracods, and could be important for evaluation of the history of sexual dimorphism and the origin of sex in ostracods since the early Palaeozoic. To clarify the long-term history of evolutionary processes in terms of their ecology and reproductive modes since the Ordovician, more data on sexual dimorphism of ostracod carapaces with appendages of many taxa that exhibit heterochronic morphology should be collected.
3. Many examples of ostracod sexual dimorphism are found in various taxonomic groups, including both living and extinct species. However, the actual functions of most of the dimorphic characteristics remain unclear, even for many living species, although many hypotheses have been put forward. Many of these sexually dimorphic characteristics are likely strongly related to the ecology of reproductive modes, such as mating behaviour and brood care. To clarify the actual functions in living species, ostracod behaviour, especially mating and brood care under breeding conditions, should be observed using video recordings. The lack of such observations is the primary reason why the ecological behaviour of most living ostracod species is unclear.

4. To elucidate the functions of sexually dimorphic characteristics in extinct groups; *e.g.*, the brood pouch of Palaeocopida in the Palaeozoic, fossil eggs or juvenile carapaces in the inner part of the adult carapaces from Palaeozoic sediments must be identified. For Palaeocopida, we must attempt to find fossils resting their appendages, despite their rarity. Furthermore, detailed observation of the ecological behaviour of living species will facilitate understanding of the actual functions of sexually dimorphic morphology in both living and extinct species [31]. Due to the excellent ostracod fossil record from Palaeozoic to Cenozoic, the living ostracod sexual dimorphism data can be applied to extinct species. Combined studies of the ecology and functional morphology of both living and fossil ostracod species will clarify the history of the evolutionary ecology and reproductive modes of organisms during the last ca. 500 million years.

Author details

Hirokazu Ozawa
Earth Sciences Laboratory, College of Bioresource Sciences, Nihon University, Fujisawa, Kanagawa, Japan

Acknowledgement

I wish to thank Y. Tanimura (National Museum of Nature and Science, Japan) for kind assistance of preparing the manuscript in various aspects. Thanks are also due to T. Kamiya, S. Tsukawaki, M. Kato, T. Ishii, T. Sato (Kanazawa University), A. Tsukagoshi, S. Yamada (Shizuoka University), R. J. Smith (Lake Biwa Museum), R. M. Karasz (Ludwig-Maximilians-University), T. Irizuki (Shimane University), H. Takata (Pusan University), B. C. Zhou (Shanghai Museum of Natural History), K. Ikehara, H. Katayama (AIST, Japan), H. Domitsu (University of Shiga Prefecture), A. Nojo (Hokkaido University of Education), P. J. Hayward (University of Wales Swansea) and the late N. Ikeya, Y. Kuwano and T. Matsuzaka for many valuable suggestions for ostracod resraches, with help of various aspect for my investigation. I express my gratitude to captain, all crew of the *Tansei-maru* (JAMSTEC, Japan) and *Hakurei-maru* (AIST, Japan) and all onboard scientists for their help of collecting sediment samples during Cruises KT95-14, KT96-17, KT97-15, KT98-17, KT99-14, KT00-14, KT01-14, KT04-20 and GH98. Thanks are also due to R. J. Smith permitting for using figures of his literature, and to two anonymous reviwers of native English speakers for correcting my manuscript carefully.

6. References

[1] Butlin RK., Schön I., Griffiths HI. Chapter 1: Intoroduction to reproductive modes. In: Martens K. (ed.) Sex and Parthenogenesis: Evolutionary Ecology of Reproductive Modes in Non-Marine Ostracods. Leiden: Backhuys Publishers; 1998, p. 1–24.

[2] Kamiya T. Different sex-ratios in two Recent species of *Loxoconcha* (Ostracoda). Senckenbergiana Lethaia, 1998, 68: 337–345.

[3] Martens K. Preface: To mate or not to mate !. In: Martens K. (ed.) Sex and Parthenogenesis: Evolutionary Ecology of Reproductive Modes in Non-Marine Ostracods. Leiden: Backhuys Publishers; 1998, p. xv–xvii.

[4] Benson RH., Berdan JM., van den Bold WA., Hanai T., Hessland I., Howe HV., Kesling RV., Levinson SA., Reyment RA., Moore RC., Scott HW., Shaver RH., Sohn IG., Stover LE., Swain FM., Sylvester–Bradley PC. Treatise of Invertebrate Palaeontology, Part Q Arthropoda 3, Crustacea, Ostracoda. New York: Geological Society of America, Boulder: University of Kansas Press; 1961.

[5] Benson RH. The ontogeny of an ostracodologist. The Paleontological Society Papers, 2003, 9: 1–8.

[6] Ozawa H. Chapter 4.1.8: Ostracoda. In: Tanimura Y., Tuji A. (eds.) Microfossils: Their microscopic world explored. A Book Series from the National Museum of Nature and Science 13. Hadano: Tokai University Press; 2012, p. 142–151. (in Japanese)

[7] Horne DJ. Key events in the ecological radiation of the Ostracoda. The Paleontological Society Papers, 2003, 9: 181–202.

[8] Abe K. Population structure of *Keijella bisanensis* (Okubo) (Ostracoda, Crustacea)—An inquiry into how far the population structure will be preserved in the fossil record. Journal of the Faculty of Science, University of Tokyo, Section II, 1983, 20: 443–488.

[9] Kamiya T. Heterochronic dimorphism of *Loxoconcha uranouchiensis* (Ostracoda) and its implication for speciation. Paleobiology, 1992, 18: 221–236.

[10] Horne DJ., Cohen A., Martens K. Taxonomy, morphology and biology of Quaternary and living Ostracoda. In: Holmes JA., Chivas A. (eds.) The Ostracoda: Applications in Quaternary Research, AGU Geophysical Monograph Series 131. Washington DC.: America Geophysical Union; 2002, p. 5–36.

[11] Clarkson ENK. Invertebrate Palaeontology and Evolution (4th Edition). Oxford: Blackwell Science; 1998.

[12] Callomon JH. Sexual dimorphism in Jurassic ammonites. Transactions of the Leicester Literary and Philosophical Society, 1963, 57: 21–56.

[13] Makowski H. Problem of sexual dimorphism in ammonites. Palaeontologia Polonica, 1963, 12: 1–92.

[14] Maeda H. Dimorphism of Late Cretaceous false-puzosine ammonites, *Yokoyamaceras* Wright and Matsumoto, 1954 and *Neopuzosua* Matsumoto, 1954. Transactions and Proceedings of Palaeontological Society of Japan, New Series, 1993, 170: 186–211.

[15] Yajima M., Kamiya T. Chapter 1: Reproduction (Sex ratio & Sexual dimorphism). In: Ikeya N., Tanabe K. (eds.) Life-History of Paleontology, Paleontological Science Series 3. Tokyo: Asakura Publishing; 2001, p. 1–8. (in Japanese)

[16] Ozawa H., Ishii T. Taxonomy and sexual dimorphism of a new species of *Loxoconcha* (Podocopida: Ostracoda) from the Pleistocene of the Japan Sea. Zoological Journal of the Linnean Society, 2008, 153: 239–251.

[17] Smith RJ., Kamiya T., Horne DJ. Living males of the 'ancient asexual' Darwinulidae (Ostracoda: Crustacea). Proceedings of the Royal Society B, 2006, 273: 1569–1578.

[18] Tsukagoshi A. Species diversity and paleontology: an example of interstitial Ostracoda. Fossils (Palaeontolological Society of Japan), 2004, 75: 18–23. (in Japanese with English abstract)

[19] Tsukagoshi A. Chapter 2: Geobiological history perused by researches for Ostracoda. In: Katakura H., Mawatari S. (eds.) Diversity of Organisms, Organism Science in the 21th Century Series 2. Tokyo: Baifukan; 2007, p. 37–70. (in Japanese)

[20] Athersuch J., Horne DJ., Whittaker JE. Marine and brackish water ostracods. Synopsis of the British Fauna (New Series) 43. Leiden: EJ. Brill; 1989.

[21] Tsukagoshi A. Ontogenetic change of distributional patterns of pore systems in *Cythere* species and its phylogenetic significance. Lethaia, 1990; 23: 225–241.

[22] Tsukagoshi A. Recommendations from paleontology: fossils that demonstrate organismal phylogeny. In: Iwatsuki K., Mawatari S. (eds.) Species Diversity, Biodiversity Series. Tokyo: Shokabo; 1996, p. 173–187.(in Japanese)

[23] Siveter DJ., Sutton MD., Briggs DEG., Siveter DJ. An ostracode crustacean with soft parts from the Lower Silurian. Science, 2003, 300: 1749–1751.

[24] Tsukagoshi A., Ikeya N. The ostracod genus *Cythere* O. F. Müller, 1785 and its species. Transactions and Proceedings of the Palaeontological Society of Japan, New Series, 1987, 148: 197–222.

[25] Horne DJ., Danielopol DL., Martens K. Chapter 10: Reproductive behaviour. In: Martens K. (ed.) Sex and Parthenogenesis: Evolutionary Ecology of Reproductive Modes in Non-Marine Ostracods. Leiden: Backhuys Publishers; 1998, p. 157–195.

[26] Sato T., Kamiya T. Taxonomy and geographical distribution of recent *Xestoleberis* species (Cytheroidea, Ostracoda, Crustacea) from Japan. Paleontological Research, 2007, 11: 183–227.

[27] Boomer I., Horne DJ., Slipper IJ. The use of ostracodes in paleoenvironmental studies or what can you do with an ostracode shell? The Paleontological Society Papers, 2003, 9: 153–179.

[28] Cronin TM., Dwyer GS. Deep-sea ostracodes and climate change. The Paleontological Society Papers, 2003, 9: 247–264.

[29] Ozawa H. Chapter 2: Extinction of Cytheroidean ostracodes (Crustacea) in shallow-water around Japan in relation to environmental fluctuations since the early Pleistocene. In: Tepper GH. (ed.) Species Diversity and Extinction. New York: Nova Science Publishers, Incorporation; 2010, p. 61–109.

[30] Abe K., Vannier J. Mating behavior in the podocopid ostracode *Bicornucythere bisanensis* (Okubo, 1975): rotation of a female by a male with asymmetric fifth limbs. Journal of Crustacean Biology, 1991, 11: 250–260.

[31] Kesling RV. Copulatory adaptations in ostracods Part III. Adaptations in some extinct ostracods. Contributions from the Museum of Paleontology, The University of Michigan, 1969, 22: 273–312.

[32] Hanai T. Cretaceous non-marine Ostracoda from the Sungai Group in Manchuria. Journal of Faculty of Sciences, University of Tokyo, Section II, 1951, 7: 403–430.
[33] Ozawa H., Kamiya T. Taxonomy and palaeobiogeographical significance for four new species of *Semicytherura* (Ostracoda, Crustacea) from the Early Pleistocene Omma Formation at the Japan Sea coast. Journal of Micropalaeontology, 2008, 27: 135–146.
[34] Okada Y. Stratigraphy and Ostracoda from the Late Cenozoic strata of the Oga Peninsula, Akita Prefecture. Transactions and Proceedings of the Palaeontological Society of Japan, New Series, 1979, 115: 143–173.
[35] Nakao Y., Tsukagoshi A. Brackish-water Ostracoda (Crustacea) from the Obitsu River Estuary, central Japan. Species Diversity, 2002, 7: 67–115.
[36] Ozawa H., Kamiya T. A new species of *Aurila* (Crustacea: Ostracoda: Cytheroidea: Hemicytheridae) from the Pleistocene Omma Formation on the coast of the Sea of Japan. Species Diversity, 2009, 14: 27–39.
[37] Ikeya N., Abe K. Natural History of the Ostracoda. Tokyo: University of Tokyo Presss; 1996. (in Japanese)
[38] Ozawa H. Middle Pleistocene ostracods from the Naganuma Formation in the Sagami Group, Kanagawa Prefecture, central Japan: palaeo-biogeographical significance of the bay fauna in Northwest Pacific margin. Paleontological Research, 2009, 13: 231–244.
[39] Smith RJ., Hiruta S. A new species of *Metacypris* (Limnocytherinae, Cytheroidea, Ostracoda, Crustacea) from Hokkaido, Japan. Species Diversity, 2004, 9: 37–46.
[40] Ikeya N., Yamaguchi T. An Introduction to Crustacean Paleobiology (UP Biology Series 93). Tokyo: University of Tokyo Press; 1993. (in Japanese)
[41] Jaanusson V. Functional morphology of the shell in platycope ostracodes–a study of arrested evolution. Lethaia, 1985, 18: 3–84.
[42] Schram FR. Crustacea. Oxford: Oxford University Press; 1986.
[43] Tsukagoshi A. On *Callistocythere pumila* Hanai. Stereo-Atlas of Ostracod Shells, 1998, 25: 9–16.
[44] Kamiya T., Ozawa H., Obata M. Quaternary and Recent marine Ostracoda in Hokuriku district, the Japan Sea coast. In: Ikeya N. (ed.) Field Excursion Guidebook of the 14th International Symposium of Ostracoda, Shizuoka. Shizuoka: Organising Committee of 14th ISO; 2001, p. 73–106.
[45] Okubo I. *Callistocythere pumila*, Hanai and *Leguminocythereis bisanensis* sp. nov. in the Inland Sea, Japan (Ostracoda). Proceedings of Japanese Society of Systematic Zoology, 1975, 11: 23–31.
[46] Okubo I. Five Species of *Callistocythere* (Ostracoda) from the Inland Sea of Seto. Researches on Crustacea (Carcinologic Society of Japan), 1979, 9: 13–25.
[47] Ikeya N., Shiozaki M. Characteristic of the inner-bay ostracodes around the Japanese Islands–the use of ostracodes to reconstruct paleoenvironments. Memoirs of the Geological Society of Japan, 1993, 39: 15–32. (in Japanese with English abstract)

[48] Kajiyama E. The Ostracoda from Misaki, part 3, Zoological Magazine of Tokyo (Doubutsugaku-zassi), 1913, 25: 1–16. (in Japanese)

[49] Schornikov EI., Schaitanov SV. A new genus of ostracods from Fareastern seas. Biologiya Morya, 1979, 2: 48–54. (in Russian)

[50] Abe K., Vannier J. The role of 5th limbs in mating behavior of two marine podocopid ostracods, *Bicornucythere bisanensis* (Okubo, 1975) and *Xestoleberis hanaii* Ishizaki, 1968. In: Mckenzie KG., Jones PJ. (eds.) Ostracoda in the Earth and Life Sciences. Rotterdam: AA. Balkema; 1993, p. 581–590.

[51] Vannier J., Abe K. Functional morphology and behavior of *Vargula hilgendorfi* (Ostracoda: Myodocopida) from Japan, and discussion of its crustacean ectoparasite: preliminary results from video recordings. Journal of Crustacean Biology, 1993, 13: 51–76.

[52] Athersuch J., Horne, DJ. A Review of some European genera of the Family Loxoconchidae (Crustacea: Ostracoda). Zoological Journal of the Linnean Society, 1984, 81: 1–22.

[53] Hanai T., Ikeya N., Yajima M. Checklist of Ostracoda from Southest Asia. University Museum, University of Tokyo Bulletin, 1980, 17: 1–236.

[54] Tanaka G., Ikeya N. Migration and speciation of the *Loxoconcha japonica* species group (Ostracoda) in East Asia. Paleontological Research, 2002, 6: 265–284.

[55] Ishizaki K. Ostracodes from Uranouchi Bay, Kochi Prefecture, Japan. Tohoku University, Science Report, 2nd Series (Geology), 1968, 40: 1–45.

[56] Hanai T., Ikeya N., Ishizaki K., Sekiguchi Y., Yajima M. Checklist of Ostracoda from Japan and its adjacent seas. University Museum, University of Tokyo Bulletin, 1977, 12: 1–119.

[57] Zhou BC. Recent ostracode fauna in the Pacific off Southwest Japan. Memoirs of Faculty of Science, Kyoto University, Series of Geology & Mineralogy, 1995, 57: 21–98.

[58] Tsukawaki S., Ozawa H., Domitsu H., Kamiya T., Kato M., Oda M. Preliminary results from the R.V. *Tansei-maru* Cruise KT98-17 in the southwestern marginal Part of the Japan Sea–Sediments, Benthic and Planktonic Foraminifers, and Ostracodes. Bulletin of the Japan Sea Research Institute, 2000, 31: 89–119.

[59] Irizuki T. Fossil Ostracoda from the lower Pleistocene Masuda Formation, Tanega-shima Island, southern Japan. Geoscience Reports of Shimane University, 2004, 23: 65–77.

[60] Ikeya N., Tanaka G., Tsukagoshi A. Ostracoda. Palaeontological Society of Japan, Special Papers, 2003, 41: 37–131.

[61] Kamiya T. Phylogenetics estimated from fossil information–the pore systems of Ostracoda. Iden (Genetics), 1997, 51: 28–34. (in Japanese).

[62] Irizuki T. Morphology and taxonomy of some Japanese hemicytherin Ostracoda–with particular reference to ontogenetic changes of marginal pores. Transactions and Proceedings of Palaeontological Society of Japan, New Series, 1993, 170: 186–211.

[63] Ishii T., Kamiya T., Tsukagoshi A. Phylogeny and evolution of *Loxoconcha* (Ostracoda, Crustacea) species around Japan. Hydrobiologia, 2005, 538: 81–94.

[64] Smith RJ., Kamiya, T. The ontogeny of the entocytherid ostracod *Uncinocythere occidentalis* (Kozloff & Whitman, 1954) Hart, 1962 (Crustacea). Hydrobiologia, 2005, 538: 217–229.

[65] Benson RH., Coleman-II GL. Recent marine ostracodes from the eastern Gulf of Mexico. The University of Kansas Paleontological Contributions, Arthropoda Article, 1963, 2: 1–52.

[66] Ishizaki K. Ostracodes from Aomori Bay, Aomori Prefecture, Northeast Honshu, Japan. Tohoku University, Science Report, 2nd Series (Geology), 1971, 43: 59–97.

[67] Nagamori H., Furukawa R., Hayatsu K. Geology of the Togakushi district. Quadrangle Series, 1: 50,000. Tsukuba: Geological Survey of Japan, AIST; 2003. (in Japanese with English abstract)

[68] Motoyama I., Nagamori H. Radiolarians from the Pliocene of the Hokushin district, Nagano Prefecture, Japan. Journal of Geological Society of Japan, 2006, 112: 541–548. (in Japanese with English abstract)

[69] Irizuki T., Kusumoto M., Ishida K., Tanaka Y. Sea-level changes and water structures between 3.5 and 2.8 Ma in the central part of the Japan Sea Borderland: Analyses of fossil Ostracoda from the Pliocene Kuwae Formation, central Japan. Palaeogeography, Palaeoclimatology, Palaeoecology, 2007, 245: 421–443.

[70] Kato M., Akada K. Takayama T., Goto T., Sato T., Kudo T., Kameo K. Calcareous microfossil biostratigraphy of the uppermost Cenozoic Formation distributed in the coast of the Japan Sea–"Sawane Formation". Annals of Science of Kanazawa University, 1995, 32: 21–38. (in Japanese)

[71] Takata H. Paleoenvironmental changes during the deposition of the Omma Formation (late Pliocene to early Pleistocene) in Oyabe area, Toyama Prefecture based on the analysis of benthic and planktonic foraminiferal assemblages. Fossils (Palaeontological Society of Japan), 2000, 67: 1–18. (in Japanese with English abstract).

[72] Okubo I. Taxonomic studies on Recent marine podocopid Ostracoda from the Inland Sea of Seto. Publications of Seto Marine Biological Laboratory, 1980, 25: 389–443.

[73] McNamara KJ. A guide to the nomenclature of heterochrony. Journal of Paleontology, 1986, 60: 4–13.

[74] McNamara KJ. Chapter 3: The role of heterochrony in evolutionary trends. In: McNamara KJ. (ed.) Evolutionary Trends. London: Belhaven Press; 1990, p. 59–74.

[75] Tsukagoshi A. Natural history of the brackish-water ostracode genus *Ishizakiella* from East Asia: evidence for heterochrony. Journal of Crustacean Biology, 1994, 14: 295–313.

[76] Tsukagoshi A., Kamiya T. Heterochrony of the ostracod hingement and its significance for taxonomy. Biological Journal of the Linnean Society, 1996, 57: 343–370.

[77] Kamiya T. Morphological and ethological adaptations of Ostracoda to microhabitats in *Zostera* beds. In: Hanai T., Ikeya N., Ishizaki K. (eds.) Evolutionary Biology of Ostracoda–Its fundamentals and applications. Tokyo: Kodansha, Amsterdam: Elsevier; 1988, p. 303–318.

Chapter 5

Sexual Dimorphism in Monoamine Metabolism in BrdU-Treated Rats Showing Behavioral Dopamine Hypersensitivity: An Animal Model of Schizophrenia

Katsumasa Muneoka and Makiko Kuwagata

Additional information is available at the end of the chapter

http://dx.doi.org/10.5772/55348

1. Introduction

A nucleotide analog 5-bromo-2′-deoxyuridine (BrdU) is a genotoxic compound that is incorporated into DNA [1]. When rodent fetuses are exposed to BrdU prenatally, the cortical development is profoundly affected. Cortical abnormalities induced by prenatal BrdU are shown as a reduction in thickness of the cerebral cortex [2]. An induction of apoptotic cell death in the mouse and rat fetal brain [3, 4] and disturbance to normal migration that induces abnormal composition of cortical glutamatergic or GABAergic neurons have been demonstrated [4]. Mouse data suggest that the prenatal BrdU treatment induced apoptotic phenomenon without sex difference (Figure 1).

Adult rats that were prenatally treated with BrdU show locomotor hyperactivity. The hyperactivity was observed in both male and female rats and was characterized as an increase in spontaneous motor activity during dark cycles observed in home cages [5] and novelty-induced hyperlocomotion in the open-field [5 - 8]. This abnormal behavior is exacerbated by the treatment with dopamine (DA) agonist, methylphenidate, which indicates that animals acquired hypersensitivity to dopaminergic stimuli [5, 8]. Recently proposed animal models for schizophrenia that knock-out candidate genes for this disease, such as neurotensin receptors [9] or calcium/calmodulin-dependent kinase II alpha [10], show hyperactive phenotypes and abnormal striatal DA function while mice overexpressing DA D_2 receptors in the striatum show unaltered locomotor activity [11]. In a major psychiatric disorder schizophrenia, disturbance in cortical development and subcortical dopaminergic abnormality have been proposed [12] and they induces hypothetical pathology in this disease "a prefrontal hypodopaminergia and a subcortical hyperdopaminergia" [13]. We propose that prenatal BrdU-treated rats is an animal model of schizophrenia based on findings that 1) the malformation of the cerebral cortex and 2) DA hypersensitivity.

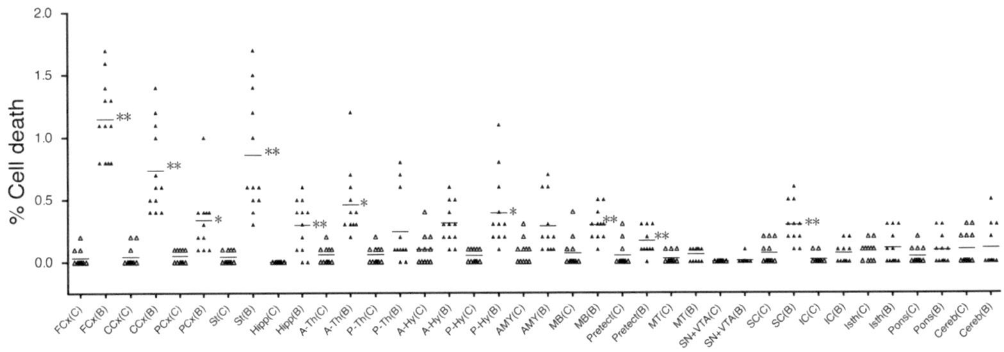

Figure 1. Incidence of cell death in fetal mouse brains on the embryonic day 12 after the treatment with BrdU at the embryonic day 11 without indenfying sex. Apoptotic features were inspected under Nissl stain. Data were indicated as percents of numbers of apoptotic cells; C and B in parentheses indicates control and BrdU-treated animals. Horizontal bars indicate means. Significant increases in the numbers of apoptotic cell death were indicated as asterisks: *, **; $P < 0.05$, 0.01, respectively vs. controls. Results suggest that apoptotic cell death occurred similarly in fetal brains between males and females because values in % cell death in BrdU-treated brains in sample of mixed males and females scattered without clustering. FCx, the frontal cortex; CCx, the central cortex; PCx, the posterior cortex; St, the striatum; Hipp, the hippocmpus; A-Th, the anterior thalamus; P-Th, the posterior thalamus; A-Hy, the anterior hypothalamus; P-Hy, the posterior thalamus; AMY, the amygdala; MB, the mamillary body; Pretect, the pretectum; MT, the mecencephalic tegmentum; SN+VTA; The sunbtantia nigra + the ventral tegmental area; SC, the superior colliculus; IC; the inferior colliculus; Isth, the inthmus; Cereb, the cerebellum.

Sexual dimorphism in animal models of mental disorders is interested theme to be explored because sexual difference has been reported in clinical features in such disorders including schizophrenia. Emergence of abnormal symptoms in human mental illnesses has been known to be relevant to the beginning of puberty and this phenomenon appears to be influenced by gonadal hormones [14]. Gender differences in the age-of-onset and prevalence of mental disorders indicate an involvement of sex hormones in schizophrenia. Schizophrenia is more likely to emerge during adolescence or shortly afterwards and the first symptoms of schizophrenia emerge earlier in men than women [15]. This is more direct evidence for the involvement of sex steroids is the observation that adult women with schizophrenia have worse psychiatric symptoms and increased rate of relapse when estrogen levels are low in premenstrual period, postparturition or postmenopausal period [16]. Furthermore, estrogen has been shown to improve recovery from acute psychotic symptoms and to reduce both positive and negative symptoms of schizophrenia [17]. In adult males with schizophrenia testosterone levels are reduced and are inversely correlated with negative symptoms [18]. Altered expression of estrogen receptor alpha putatively rendering them sex-steroid unresponsive or insensitive has been reported [19]. Blunted sex steroid signaling has implications for both males and females with schizophrenia, as testosterone can be converted directly into estrogen by brain aromatase and the lack of functional estrogen receptors is found in both males and females with schizophrenia.

The changes in hormone levels that accompany sexual maturation in puberty are critically involved in the development of the monoaminergic system [20]. In animal studies, in addition to the well-known modulatory effects of estrogen or progesterone on DA neurotransmission or DA-related behavior [21 - 25], it has been reported that neuronal systems whose dysfunction mediates the emergence of psychotic-like behavior develops after the emergence of puberty, suggesting a role for gonadal hormones in the expression of pathological phenotypes [26, 27]. A study of rhesus macaques has demonstrated that intact adult animals display attenuated prepulse inhibition than animals given prepubertal castration [28]. In addition, results from studies of sexual dimorphic effects of prenatal stress in rats imply that the developing brain of female fetuses is less sensitive to maternal stress exposure than male ones, however, enhanced aggressive behavior or disturbed estrous cycle are observed [29]. Neonatal stress manipulation, maternal deprivation from pups, increases DA and 5-HT levels in the striatum in adulthood and the magnitude of changes are greater in males than females [30].

In this chapter, we introduce the development of this animal model, their behavioral and neurochemical characters. Then, we evaluate recent obtained data of sexual dimorphic changes in DA and serotonin (5-HT) metabolisms in the prenatally BrdU-treated rats, and effects of gonadectomy that was performed during the prepubertal period.

2. Methods

2.1. Animals, drug treatments and gonadectomy

Sprague-Dawley rats were purchased from Charles River Laboratories (Tsukuba, Japan). They were housed in metal cages in a room in which the temperature and relative humidity were controlled at 24 ± 1°C and 50 ± 5%, respectively. Lights were turned on from 0700 to 1900 h daily, and food and tap water were freely accessed. At 11 weeks of age, female rats were cohabited overnight with males. Females with sperm in their vaginal smears were regarded as pregnant, and were randomly assigned to the control or test groups. The day when the insemination was confirmed was designated as GD 0. BrdU (Sigma, St. Louis, MO) was suspended in 0.5% sodium carboxymethyl cellulose (CMC Na) and intraperitoneally administered to the test animals at 1300 h daily on GD 9 through 15. Females in the test group received a BrdU dose of 50 mg/kg, whereas control females subjected to the same regime received 0.5% CMC Na (5 ml/kg). The dosages were based on body weight on GD 9. The day of birth was designated postnatal day 0 (PND 0). On PND 1, each litter was reduced to eight animals; four males and four females. On PND 21, all offspring were weaned. At 10 weeks of age, one male and female animal obtained from an independent litter were sacrificed by decapitation and their brains were removed between 1600 and 1800 h. Each brain was subsequently dissected on ice. All tissues were stored at –80°C until the assay. We arranged other groups to investigate the effect of gonadectomy: the BrdU/GDX and BrdU/non-GDX groups. Female pups obtained from BrdU-treated pregnant rats were used for this investigation. Female offspring assigned to the BrdU/GDX group were gonadectomized at 21 days of age, while animals assigned to the BrdU/non-GDX group received a sham operation.

2.2. Biochemical measurements

DA, 5-HT and their major metabolites, dihydroxyphenylacetic acid (DOPAC), homovanilic acid (HVA), and 5-hydroxy-3-indolacetic acid (5-HIAA) were determined by reversephase high-performance liquid chromatography with electrochemical detection (HPLC-ECD) as previously described [31]. Briefly, the brain tissues were homogenized in 0.1 M perchloric acid containing 1 mM EDTA and 2 mM $Na_2S_2O_5$. Chloroform was added, and the mixture was then centrifuged at 11752 x *g* for 30 min at 4°C. The supernatant was removed and injected into the HPLC system. The HPLC system consisted of an EP-300 pump (Eicom Co., Kyoto, Japan), an ODS C18 reverse-phase column (Eicompak MA-5ODS, 4.5• x 150 mm; Eicom Co.) and an ECD-300 electrochemical detector (Eicom Co.) with a graphite working electrode maintained at +0.7 V with respect to an Ag/AgCl reference electrode. The mobile phase was 0.035 M sodium acetate–0.05 M citric acid (pH=3.9) containing 1.1 mM octanesulfonate, 8.3 mM EDTA, and 15% methanol (v/v). As indices of DA turnovers, DOPAC/DA and HVA/DA ratios were calculated. As an index of 5-HT turnover, 5-HIAA/5-HT ratio was calculated.

2.3. Evaluation of sexual behavior in offsprings

At 15 weeks of age, male animals were presented with an ovariectomized female brought into sexual receptivity by sequential treatment with estradiol benzoate and followed progesterone. Musculine sexual behavior was evaluated in the numbers of mounts and latency to the first mount. After this observation, each male was cohabited with an treated female to evaluate fertility.

2.4. Statistical analysis

Data are shown as means ± S.E.M. Student's *t*-tests and one-way ANOVA were applied for comparisons between two groups and three groups, respectively. Monoamine contents were formulated into percent values of controls before analysis for differences between Male-BrdU, Female-BrdU and Female-BrdU-GDX because each group had independent controls. Post-hoc Tukey/Kramer tests was performed accompanied with one-way ANOVAs. Two-way ANOVAs were applied to analyze two independent factors (Sex and BrdU) simultaneously. *P* values less than 0.05 were considered to be statistically significant.

3. Results

3.1. Behavioral and pharmacological aspects of prenatally BrdU-treated rats

Behavioral and pharmacological aspects of prenatally BrdU-treated rats are summarized in Table 1. Spontaneous locomotor activity in the open-field was elevated both in male and female BrdU-treated rats when it was measured for 3 and 60 min [5, 8]. Activity in home cages of BrdU-treated animals was also elevated both in males and females but this hyperactivity was found in the dark cycle but not in the light cycle. The characteristic hyperactivity in the open-field induced by prenatal BrdU treatment was challenged to be influenced with dopaminergic, serotonergic and noradrenergic agents; methylphenidate (DA agonist), SCH23390 (DA D_1 receptor antagonist), sulpiride (DA D_2 receptor antagonist), NAN190 (5-HT_{1A} receptor antagonist), ketanserin (5-HT_{2A} receptor antagonist), paroxetine (selective serotonin reuptake inhibitor) and desipramine (noradrenaline reuptake inhibitor) [5, 6]. The data were obtained in male rats. Methylphenidate facilitated hyperlocomotion shown in BrdU-treated rats dose-dependently. The dose of methylphenidate (1 mg/kg) that did not stimulate locomotion in controls elevated locomotor activity of BrdU-treated rats [5, 8]. SCH23390 and NAN190 decreased activity in BrdU-treated rats but similar changes were also found in control rats. Effects of sulpiride and ketanserin on hyperactivity of the BrdU-treated rats were not certain. However, paroxetine and desipramine suppressed hyperlocomotion of BrdU-treated rats dose-dependently without influencing the activity of controls [5]. These results suggest that BrdU exposed to fetus induced similar behavioral phenotype in male and female animals. The BrdU-treated animals seem to show behavioral hypersensitivity to a DA agonist. Inhibition of reuptake of 5-HT or noradrenaline seems to suppress locomotor activity specifically in BrdU-treated rats rather than antagonists to DA or 5-HT receptors.

	Male	Female
Spontaneous locomotor activity		
Open field test (3 min)	↑	↑
Open field test (60 min)	↑	↑
Activity in home cages (light cycle)	→	→
Activity in home cages (dark cycle)	↑	↑
Effects of pharmacological challenges on BrdU-induced hyperactivity (data obtained from male rats)		
Methylphenidate (dopamine agonist)	↑	
SCH23390 (dopamine D_1 receptor antagonist)	↓	
Sulpiride (dopamine D_2 receptor antagonist)	→ or ↑	
NAN190 (5-HT_{1A} receptor antagonist)	↓	
Ketanserin (5-HT_{2A} receptor antagonist)	→	
Paroxetine (selective serotonin reuptake inhibitor)	↓	
Desipramine (noradrenaline reuptake inhibitor)	↓	

Table 1. Behavioral and pharmacological aspects of prenatally BrdU-treated rats

3.2. Effects of prenatal BrdU treatment on DA and 5-HT and their metabolites in male and female offsprings

In the frontal cortex, brain contents of 5-HT and 5-HIAA seem to elevate in BrdU-treated females but not in BrdU-treated males (Figure 2A). In the striatum, DA and DOPAC contents significantly decreased in BrdU-treated males while DA contents significantly elevated and DOPAC contents showed control levels in BrdU-treated females (Figure 2B).

BrdU-treated male rats shows prominent increases in striatal 5-HT and 5-HIAA while 5-HT levels were mildly elevated and 5-HIAA levels were comparable to controls' values in BrdU-treated females (Figure 2B). Significant reductions in DA and a significant reduction and a tendency to decrease in DOPAC contents were found in the hypothalamus of male and female BrdU-treated rats (Figure 2C). There were a significant reduction in HVA in females and a significant reduction in 5-HIAA in males in BrdU-treated animals in the midbrain (Figure 2D).

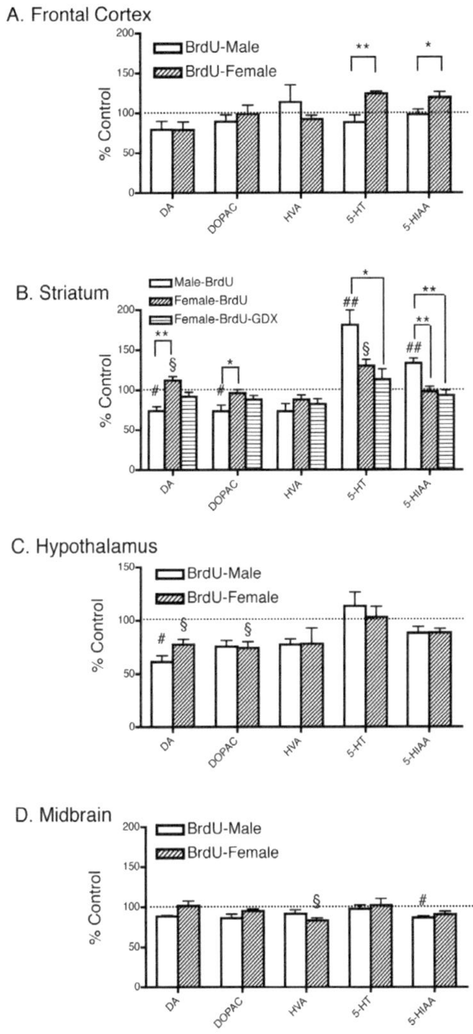

Figure 2. Changes in tissue contents of monoamines and their metabolites in prenatally BrdU-treated rats. Data are indicated as percent values of controls. Statistical significance in difference between controls and BrdU-treated animals is indicated as symbols located at the top of columns; #, $P < 0.05$ vs. male controls; ##, $P < 0.01$ vs. male controls; §, $P < 0.05$ vs. female controls. Statistical significance in percent values between BrdU-treated males (Male-BrdU), BrdU-treated females (Female-BrdU) and BrdU-treated females that are given gonadectomy (Female-BrdU-GDX) is indicated as asterisks located between columns; *, $P < 0.05$; **, $P < 0.01$.

3.3. Effects of prenatal BrdU treatment and sex on rations of DOPAC/DA, HVA/DA and 5-HT

There was no significant effect of BrdU or Sex on DOPAC/DA, HVA/DA or 5-HT in the frontal cortex (Figure 3A). In the striatum and the midbrain, significant effects of Sex on all measured turnover ratios and a significant effect of BrdU on 5-HIAA/5-HT ratio were detected (Figure 3B and D). There were significant effects of Sex on DOPAC/DA and 5-HIAA/5-HT and a significant effect of BrdU on 5-HIAA/5-HT in the hypothalamus (Figure 3C). Significant interaction of the two independent factors Sex and BrdU was detected in any measured values. There data suggest that prenatal BrdU affects 5-HT turnovers in the striatum, hypothalamus and midbrain in male and female offsprings in same manner. These brain regions seem to show intrinsic sexual differences in DA and 5-HT turnovers.

3.4. Sexual dimorphism in the effects of prenatal BrdU treatment on DA and 5-HT metabolism

Statistical analysis indicated significant sexual dimorphic effects of prenatal BrdU on monoamines in the frontal cortex and the striatum but not in the hypothalamus and midbrain. There were significant differences in percent changes of 5-HT and 5-HIAA compared with control levels between male and female offspring in the frontal cortex (Figure 2A). In the striatum, significant differences in percent changes of DA, DOPAC and 5-HIAA compared with control levels were detected between male and female offspring in the striatum (Figure 2B).

3.5. Effects of prepubertal gonadectomy of BrdU-treated females on striatal monoamines

Results were summarized in Table 2. No statistical difference in DA and DOPAC levels were found in the BrdU-treated females that gave gonadectomy prepubertally compared with the BruU-treated male and female rats without gonadectomy although marked differences in BrdU-induced changes were found in DA and DOPAC levels between male and female groups (Figure 2B). Significant differences in 5-HT and 5-HIAA levels were found in the BrdU-treated females with gonadectomy compared with the BrdU-treated males (Figure 2B), which were similar changes to the BrdU-treated females without gonadectomy. These results indicate abolishment of sexual dimorphism by prepubertal gonadectomy in effects of prenatal BrdU treatment on the DA system but not in the 5-HT system in the striatum.

3.6. Disruption of sexual behavior in male offsprings from BrdU-treated dams

Males in the BrdU group showed the significantly lowered number of mounts and aberrant latency of the first amount, which resulted in a significant decrease in the copulation and fertility [7].

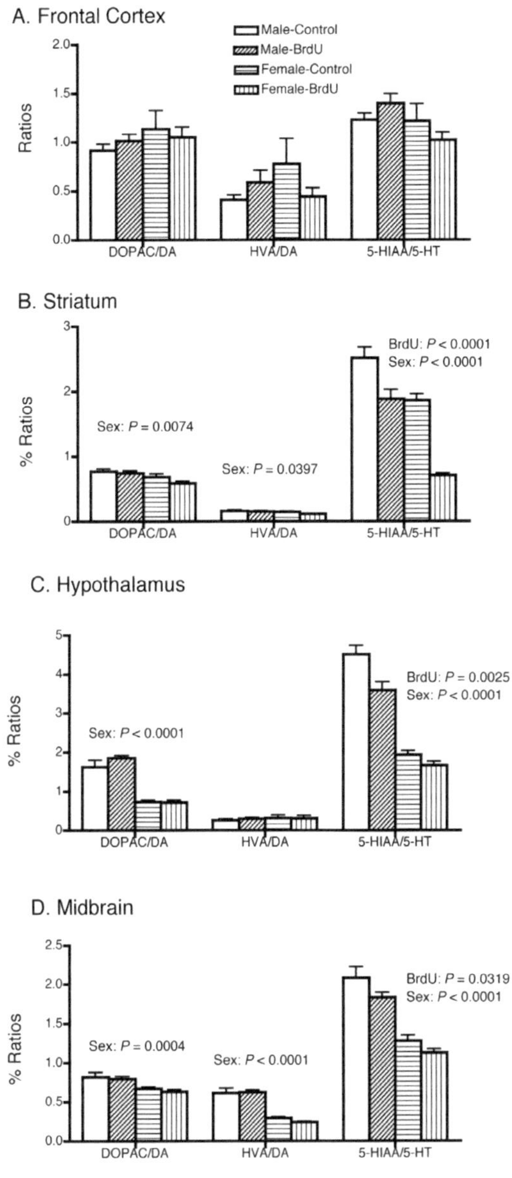

Figure 3. DOPAC/DA, HVA/DA and 5-HIAA/5-HT ratios in male controls (Male-Control), BrdU-treated males (Male-BrdU), female controls (Female-Control) and BrdU-treated females (Female-BrdU). *P* values in applied two-way ANOVAs as factors of SEX and BrdU are incorporated in figures when results were statistically significant.

Monoamines and metabolites	Male-BrdU	Female-BrdU	Female-BrdU + prepubertal gonadectomy
DA	↓↓	↑	→
DOPAC	↓↓	→	→
HVA	→	→	→
5-HT	↑↑	↑	→
5-HIAA	↑↑	→	→

Table 2. A summary of sexual dimorphic effects of prenatal BrdU on the monoamine metabolism in the striatum

4. Discussion

The treatment with BrdU in the mid-pregnancy induced apoptotic cell death in fetal brains in rodents without sex difference. Offspring from prenatal BrdU-treatment showed prominent hyperactivity in familiar or novel environment after maturation, which was observed both in male and females. However, sexual behavior was disrupted in male offspring when they were prenatally treated with BrdU. In this animal model, sexual dimorphism in monoamine metabolism was revealed. Most obvious differences in monoamine metabolism between males and females were found in DA contents in the adult striatum; a decrease in males and an increase in females. While DA levels seem to be reduced in the frontal cortex similarly in males and females with prenatal BrdU treatment. Another sexual dimorphic effect was changes in 5-HT in the striatum and the frontal cortex. Increases in 5-HT were also found in the striatum in both sex but the magnitude in the changes were larger in males rather than in females. Increased 5-HT levels in the frontal cortex were obvious in females treated with BrdU prenetally but not in males. Therefore, prenatal BrdU treatment affects the striatal DA and 5-HT system most seriously in males. Effects of prenatal BrdU on the frontal cortical DA were moderate and the magnitude was similar in males and females. Cortical 5-HT was changes only in females.

Results from the study of gonadectomy during prepubertal period demonstrated that the most obvious effect this manipulation was the abolishment sexual dimorphism in the effect of prenatal BrdU treatment on striatal DA. This phenomenon suggests that female-specific hormones are necessary for the development of striatal DA function in females. Female sexual hormones seem to exert a protective effect on DA neurons. In adult rodents, less neurotoxicity of 6-OHDA on midbrain DA neurons [32] and of methamphetamine on striatal DA neurons have been reported in females compared with males [33]. Furthermore, it has been suggested that susceptibility of the striatal dopaminergic system to 6-OHDA is reduced in male rats but enhanced in female rats by gonadectomy [34]. A development study indicates that gonadal hormones in female mice during the pre-pubertal period are necessary for estrogen to exert neuroprotective effects on the nigrostriatal dopaminergic system [35]. In addition, adrenalectomy accompanied with oral corticosterone replacement reduces anxiety-like behavior in male rats but it does not have significant effects on females

[36]. A study of rhesus macaques has demonstrated that intact animals display less prepulse inhibition than animals given prepubertal castration [28]. This study also reveals that testosterone levels are correlated with tyrosine hydroxylase levels in the putamen among intact animals, suggesting the attenuation of PPI by gonadal sex hormones is mediated by dopaminergic activity in striatal regions. In addition, methamphetamine increases latent inhibition in male rats while this agent decreases this behavior in female rats, suggesting that presynaptic dopaminergic function shows a sex difference [37]. Hence, striatal DA function, especially presynaptic DA function may be different intrinsically between males and females.

The reduced DA and DOPAC in the striatum can be interpreted as a decreased total DA contents in presynaptic DA terminals that imply decrement of the number in DA presynaptic terminals or reduced DA synthesis rates. Ineffectiveness of DA receptor antagonists on hyperlocomotion found in BrdU-rats also supports abnormality in presynaptic function rather than postsynaptic DA receptors. In rodent, DA agonists usually facilitate locomotor activity. This study indicated opposite changes in striatal DA between males and females as an effect of prenatal BrdU while hyperlocomotion was obviously detected in both sex. Hence, the hyperlocomotion may be attributed to DA abnormality in the frontal cortex because the change was same in males and females.

Schizophrenia includes multiple pathology in brain functions. Striatal dysfunction is thought to be a fundamental element in schizophrenia [13]. A study using functional magnetic resonance imaging (fMRI) in schizophrenic patients has demonstrated that increased coherent intrinsic activity in the dorsal striatum during psychosis is predictive for delusion and hallucination and increased activity during psychotic remission in the ventral striatum is predictive for blunted affect and emotional withdrawal [38]. A positron emission tomography (PET) study has indicated an increased DA D_2/D_3 receptor density in a restricted area in the striatum [39]. A double-blind PET study has indicated that D_2 blockade in the striatum predicts antipsychotic response better than frontal, temporal, thalamic occupancy [40]. In addition, an involvement of the striatum in the cognitive impairment in schizophrenia has been proposed [41]. Furthermore, a study using recent molecular technique has shown that D_2 receptor overexpression in the striatum results in a functional deficit in the GABAergic system and this result suggests that the postulated deficit in GABAergic function in schizophrenia could be secondary to alterations in the striatum DA system [42].

It is hypothesized that psychosis is viewed as a process of aberrant salience [43] and a central role of DA is to mediate the salience of environmental events an internal representations [44]. A study using resting-state functional MRI has indicated increased that coherent intrinsic activity in the dorsal striatum during psychosis is predictive for delusion and hallucination, and that increased activity during psychotic remission in the ventral striatum is predictive for blunted affect and emotional withdrawal [38]. A meta-analysis of imaging studies using PET or single-photon emission computed tomography (SPECT) has indicated that the locus of the largest dopaminergic abnormality in schizophrenia is presynaptic, which affects DA synthesis capacity, baseline synaptic DA levels, and DA release although a primary target of current antipsychotic drugs is blockade of DA D_2/D_3 receptors [45]. Higher DA concentration in the associative striatum in schizophrenia has been shown in a PET study using [^{11}C]raclopride, and this result suggests that elevated subcortical DA function adversely affect performance of the dorsolateral prefrontal cortex in patients [46]. ^{18}F-dopa uptake into the associative striatum is elevated in patients with prodromal symptoms of schizophrenia. This finding using PET indicates that DA overactivity in individuals with prodoromal psychotic symptoms [47]. This study also shows that striatal subdivision is negatively related to verbal fluency performance, but this is not the case for the limbic subdivision. Verbal fluency depends on prefrontal function [48]. The associative striatum regulates information flow to and from the prefrontal cortex [49, 50]. These findings provide a plausible mechanistic link between striatal dopaminergic dysfunction and prefrontal or executive dysfunction in schizophrenia. In addition, 5-HT_{2c} receptor antagonist increased incentive motivation in an animal model of the negative-symptoms of schizophrenia that was produced by increasing striatal-specific DA D_2 receptor density [51]. These data suggests a possibility that the primary focus of pathology of schizophrenia is the striatum, which includes abnormal presynatic DA function, accompanied GABAergic and 5-HT dysfunction and parallel existence of aberrance in the prefrontal cortical function.

Although further investigation is needed, this BrdU-animal could be a possible animal model for schizophrenia given that it includes abnormal presynaptic striatal DA function with sexual dimorphism and frontal cortical dysfunction relating to DA hypersensitivity.

Author details

Katsumasa Muneoka
Showa University School of Medicine, Department of Anatomy 1,Tokyo, Japan

Makiko Kuwagata
Hatano Research Institute, Food and Drug Safety Center, Toxicology Division, Kanagawa, Japan

5. References

[1] Morris, S. M. (1991): The genetic toxicology of 5-bromodeoxyuridine in mammalian cells. *Mutat Res*, Vol. 258, No. 2,pp.161-188, 0027-5107 (Print) 0027-5107 (Linking)

[2] Kolb, B., Pederson, B., Ballermann, M., Gibb, R.& Whishaw, I. Q. (1999): Embryonic and postnatal injections of bromodeoxyuridine produce age-dependent morphological and behavioral abnormalities. *J Neurosci*, Vol. 19, No. 6,pp.2337-2346, 0270-6474 (Print) 0270-6474 (Linking)

[3] Kuwagata, M., Ogawa, T., Nagata, T.& Shioda, S. (2007): The evaluation of early embryonic neurogenesis after exposure to the genotoxic agent 5-bromo-2'-deoxyuridine in mice. *Neurotoxicology*, Vol. 28, No. 4,pp.780-789, 0161-813X (Print) 0161-813X (Linking)

[4] Ogawa, T., Kuwagata, M., Muneoka, K. T.& Shioda, S. (2005): Neuropathological examination of fetal rat brain in the 5-bromo-2'-deoxyuridine-induced neurodevelopmental disorder model. *Congenit Anom (Kyoto)*, Vol. 45, No. 1,pp.14-20, 0914-3505 (Print) 0914-3505 (Linking)
[5] Orito, K., Morishima, A., Ogawa, T., Muneoka, K., Kuwagata, M., Takata, J., Mishima, K.& Fujiwara, M. (2009): Characteristic behavioral anomalies in rats prenatally exposed to 5-bromo-2'-deoxyuridine. *Int J Dev Neurosci*, Vol. 27, No. 1,pp.81-86, 0736-5748 (Print) 0736-5748 (Linking)
[6] Kuwagata, M., Muneoka, K. T., Ogawa, T., Takigawa, M.& Nagao, T. (2004): Locomotor hyperactivity following prenatal exposure to 5-bromo-2'-deoxyuridine: neurochemical and behavioral evidence of dopaminergic and serotonergic alterations. *Toxicol Lett*, Vol. 152, No. 1,pp.63-71, 0378-4274 (Print) 0378-4274 (Linking)
[7] Kuwagata, M.& Nagao, T. (1998): Behavior and reproductive function of rat male offspring treated prenatally with 5-bromo-2'-deoxyuridine. *Reprod Toxicol*, Vol. 12, No. 5,pp.541-549, 0890-6238 (Print) 0890-6238 (Linking)
[8] Muneoka, K., Kuwagata, M., Iwata, M., Shirayama, Y., Ogawa, T.& Takigawa, M. (2006): Dopamine transporter density and behavioral response to methylphenidate in a hyperlocomotor rat model. *Congenit Anom (Kyoto)*, Vol. 46, No. 3,pp.155-159, 0914-3505 (Print) 0914-3505 (Linking)
[9] Liang, Y., Boules, M., Li, Z., Williams, K., Miura, T., Oliveros, A.& Richelson, E. (2010): Hyperactivity of the dopaminergic system in NTS1 and NTS2 null mice. *Neuropharmacology*, Vol. 58, No. 8,pp.1199-1205, 1873-7064 (Electronic) 0028-3908 (Linking)
[10] Novak, G.& Seeman, P. (2010): Hyperactive mice show elevated D2(High) receptors, a model for schizophrenia: Calcium/calmodulin-dependent kinase II alpha knockouts. *Synapse*, Vol. 64, No. 10,pp.794-800, 1098-2396 (Electronic) 0887-4476 (Linking)
[11] Kellendonk, C., Simpson, E. H., Polan, H. J., Malleret, G., Vronskaya, S., Winiger, V., Moore, H.& Kandel, E. R. (2006): Transient and selective overexpression of dopamine D2 receptors in the striatum causes persistent abnormalities in prefrontal cortex functioning. *Neuron*, Vol. 49, No. 4,pp.603-615, 0896-6273 (Print) 0896-6273 (Linking)
[12] Carlsson, A. (1995): Neurocircuitries and neurotransmitter interactions in schizophrenia. *Int Clin Psychopharmacol*, Vol. 10 Suppl 3, pp.21-28, 0268-1315 (Print) 0268-1315 (Linking)
[13] Howes, O. D.& Kapur, S. (2009): The dopamine hypothesis of schizophrenia: version III--the final common pathway. *Schizophr Bull*, Vol. 35, No. 3,pp.549-562, 0586-7614 (Print) 0586-7614 (Linking)
[14] Goel, N.& Bale, T. L. (2009): Examining the intersection of sex and stress in modelling neuropsychiatric disorders. *J Neuroendocrinol*, Vol. 21, No. 4,pp.415-420, 1365-2826 (Electronic) 0953-8194 (Linking)
[15] Hafner, H. (2003): Gender differences in schizophrenia. *Psychoneuroendocrinology*, Vol. 28 Suppl 2, pp.17-54, 0306-4530 (Print) 0306-4530 (Linking)

[16] Seeman, M. V. (1996): Schizophrenia, gender, and affect. *Can J Psychiatry*, Vol. 41, No. 5,pp.263-264, 0706-7437 (Print) 0706-7437 (Linking)
[17] Kulkarni, J., Riedel, A., de Castella, A. R., Fitzgerald, P. B., Rolfe, T. J., Taffe, J.& Burger, H. (2001): Estrogen - a potential treatment for schizophrenia. *Schizophr Res*, Vol. 48, No. 1,pp.137-144, 0920-9964 (Print)
[18] Ko, Y. H., Jung, S. W., Joe, S. H., Lee, C. H., Jung, H. G., Jung, I. K., Kim, S. H.& Lee, M. S. (2007): Association between serum testosterone levels and the severity of negative symptoms in male patients with chronic schizophrenia. *Psychoneuroendocrinology*, Vol. 32, No. 4,pp.385-391, 0306-4530 (Print) 0306-4530 (Linking)
[19] Perlman, W. R., Webster, M. J., Kleinman, J. E.& Weickert, C. S. (2004): Reduced glucocorticoid and estrogen receptor alpha messenger ribonucleic acid levels in the amygdala of patients with major mental illness. *Biol Psychiatry*, Vol. 56, No. 11,pp.844-852, 0006-3223 (Print) 0006-3223 (Linking)
[20] Knoll, J., Miklya, I., Knoll, B.& Dallo, J. (2000): Sexual hormones terminate in the rat: the significantly enhanced catecholaminergic/serotoninergic tone in the brain characteristic to the post-weaning period. *Life Sci*, Vol. 67, No. 7,pp.765-773, 0024-3205 (Print) 0024-3205 (Linking)
[21] Arad, M.& Weiner, I. (2010): Contrasting effects of increased and decreased dopamine transmission on latent inhibition in ovariectomized rats and their modulation by 17beta-estradiol: an animal model of menopausal psychosis? *Neuropsychopharmacology*, Vol. 35, No. 7,pp.1570-1582, 1740-634X (Electronic) 0006-3223 (Linking)
[22] Callier, S., Morissette, M., Grandbois, M.& Di Paolo, T. (2000): Stereospecific prevention by 17beta-estradiol of MPTP-induced dopamine depletion in mice. *Synapse*, Vol. 37, No. 4,pp.245-251, 0887-4476 (Print) 0887-4476 (Linking)
[23] Dluzen, D. E. (2000): Neuroprotective effects of estrogen upon the nigrostriatal dopaminergic system. *J Neurocytol*, Vol. 29, No. 5-6,pp.387-399, 0300-4864 (Print) 0300-4864 (Linking)
[24] Frye, C. A.& Sora, I. (2010): Progesterone reduces hyperactivity of female and male dopamine transporter knockout mice. *Behav Brain Res*, Vol. 209, No. 1,pp.59-65, 1872-7549 (Electronic) 0166-4328 (Linking)
[25] Kuppers, E., Ivanova, T., Karolczak, M.& Beyer, C. (2000): Estrogen: a multifunctional messenger to nigrostriatal dopaminergic neurons. *J Neurocytol*, Vol. 29, No. 5-6,pp.375-385, 0300-4864 (Print) 0300-4864 (Linking)
[26] Zuckerman, L., Rimmerman, N.& Weiner, I. (2003): Latent inhibition in 35-day-old rats is not an "adult" latent inhibition: implications for neurodevelopmental models of schizophrenia. *Psychopharmacology (Berl)*, Vol. 169, No. 3-4,pp.298-307, 0033-3158 (Print) 0033-3158 (Linking)
[27] Zuckerman, L.& Weiner, I. (2003): Post-pubertal emergence of disrupted latent inhibition following prenatal immune activation. *Psychopharmacology (Berl)*, Vol. 169, No. 3-4,pp.308-313, 0033-3158 (Print) 0033-3158 (Linking)

[28] Morris, R. W., Fung, S. J., Rothmond, D. A., Richards, B., Ward, S., Noble, P. L., Woodward, R. A., Weickert, C. S.& Winslow, J. T. (2010): The effect of gonadectomy on prepulse inhibition and fear-potentiated startle in adolescent rhesus macaques. *Psychoneuroendocrinology*, Vol. 35, No. 6,pp.896-905, 1873-3360 (Electronic) 0306-4530 (Linking)

[29] Reznikov, A. G., Nosenko, N. D.& Tarasenko, L. V. (1999): Prenatal stress and glucocorticoid effects on the developing gender-related brain. *J Steroid Biochem Mol Biol*, Vol. 69, No. 1-6,pp.109-115, 0960-0760 (Print) 0960-0760 (Linking)

[30] Llorente, R., O'Shea, E., Gutierrez-Lopez, M. D., Llorente-Berzal, A., Colado, M. I.& Viveros, M. P. (2010): Sex-dependent maternal deprivation effects on brain monoamine content in adolescent rats. *Neurosci Lett*, Vol. 479, No. 2,pp.112-117, 1872-7972 (Electronic) 0304-3940 (Linking)

[31] Muneoka, K., Nakatsu, T., Fuji, T., Ogawa, T.& Takigawa, M. (1999): Prenatal administration of nicotine results in dopaminergic alteration in the neocortex. *Neurotoxicol Teratol*, Vol. 21, No. 5,pp.603-609, 0892-0362 (Print) 0892-0362 (Linking)

[32] Moroz, I. A., Rajabi, H., Rodaros, D.& Stewart, J. (2003): Effects of sex and hormonal status on astrocytic basic fibroblast growth factor-2 and tyrosine hydroxylase immunoreactivity after medial forebrain bundle 6-hydroxydopamine lesions of the midbrain dopamine neurons. *Neuroscience*, Vol. 118, No. 2,pp.463-476, 0306-4522 (Print) 0306-4522 (Linking)

[33] Dluzen, D. E., Tweed, C., Anderson, L. I.& Laping, N. J. (2003): Gender differences in methamphetamine-induced mRNA associated with neurodegeneration in the mouse nigrostriatal dopaminergic system. *Neuroendocrinol*, Vol. 77, No. 4,pp.232-238, 0028-3835 (Print) 0028-3835 (Linking)

[34] Murray, H. E., Pillai, A. V., McArthur, S. R., Razvi, N., Datla, K. P., Dexter, D. T.& Gillies, G. E. (2003): Dose- and sex-dependent effects of the neurotoxin 6-hydroxydopamine on the nigrostriatal dopaminergic pathway of adult rats: differential actions of estrogen in males and females. *Neuroscience*, Vol. 116, No. 1,pp.213-222, 0306-4522 (Print) 0306-4522 (Linking)

[35] Anderson, L. I., Leipheimer, R. E.& Dluzen, D. E. (2005): Effects of neonatal and prepubertal hormonal manipulations upon estrogen neuroprotection of the nigrostriatal dopaminergic system within female and male mice. *Neuroscience*, Vol. 130, No. 2,pp.369-382, 0306-4522 (Print) 0306-4522 (Linking)

[36] Kokras, N., Dalla, C., Sideris, A. C., Dendi, A., Mikail, H. G., Antoniou, K.& Papadopoulou-Daifoti, Z. (2012): Behavioral sexual dimorphism in models of anxiety and depression due to changes in HPA axis activity. *Neuropharmacology*, Vol. 62, No. 1,pp.436-445, 1873-7064 (Electronic) 0028-3908 (Linking)

[37] Wang, Y. C., He, B. H., Chen, C. C., Huang, A. C.& Yeh, Y. C. (2012): Gender differences in the effects of presynaptic and postsynaptic dopamine agonists on latent inhibition in rats. *Neurosci Lett*, Vol. 513, No. 2,pp.114-118, 1872-7972 (Electronic) 0304-3940 (Linking)

[38] Sorg, C., Manoliu, A., Neufang, S., Myers, N., Peters, H., Schwerthoffer, D., Scherr, M., Muhlau, M., Zimmer, C., Drzezga, A., Forstl, H., Bauml, J., Eichele, T., Wohlschlager, A. M.& Riedl, V. (2012): Increased Intrinsic Brain Activity in the Striatum Reflects Symptom Dimensions in Schizophrenia. *Schizophr Bull*, 1745-1701 (Electronic) 0586-7614 (Linking)

[39] Kegeles, L. S., Slifstein, M., Xu, X., Urban, N., Thompson, J. L., Moadel, T., Harkavy-Friedman, J. M., Gil, R., Laruelle, M.& Abi-Dargham, A. (2010): Striatal and extrastriatal dopamine D2/D3 receptors in schizophrenia evaluated with [18F]fallypride positron emission tomography. *Biol Psychiatry*, Vol. 68, No. 7,pp.634-641, 1873-2402 (Electronic) 0006-3223 (Linking)

[40] Agid, O., Mamo, D., Ginovart, N., Vitcu, I., Wilson, A. A., Zipursky, R. B.& Kapur, S. (2007): Striatal vs extrastriatal dopamine D2 receptors in antipsychotic response--a double-blind PET study in schizophrenia. *Neuropsychopharmacology*, Vol. 32, No. 6,pp.1209-1215, 0893-133X (Print) 0006-3223 (Linking)

[41] Simpson, E. H., Kellendonk, C.& Kandel, E. (2010): A possible role for the striatum in the pathogenesis of the cognitive symptoms of schizophrenia. *Neuron*, Vol. 65, No. 5,pp.585-596, 1097-4199 (Electronic) 0896-6273 (Linking)

[42] Li, Y. C., Kellendonk, C., Simpson, E. H., Kandel, E. R.& Gao, W. J. (2011): D2 receptor overexpression in the striatum leads to a deficit in inhibitory transmission and dopamine sensitivity in mouse prefrontal cortex. *Proc Natl Acad Sci U S A*, Vol. 108, No. 29,pp.12107-12112, 1091-6490 (Electronic) 0027-8424 (Linking)

[43] Howes, O. D., Egerton, A., Allan, V., McGuire, P., Stokes, P.& Kapur, S. (2009): Mechanisms underlying psychosis and antipsychotic treatment response in schizophrenia: insights from PET and SPECT imaging. *Curr Pharm Des*, Vol. 15, No. 22,pp.2550-2559, 1873-4286 (Electronic) 1381-6128 (Linking)

[44] Kapur, S. (2003): Psychosis as a state of aberrant salience: a framework linking biology, phenomenology, and pharmacology in schizophrenia. *Am J Psychiatry*, Vol. 160, No. 1,pp.13-23, 0002-953X (Print) 0002-953X (Linking)

[45] Howes, O. D., Kambeitz, J., Kim, E., Stahl, D., Slifstein, M., Abi-Dargham, A.& Kapur, S. (2012): The Nature of Dopamine Dysfunction in Schizophrenia and What This Means for Treatment: Meta-analysis of Imaging Studies. *Arch Gen Psychiatry*, Vol. 69, No. 8,pp.776-786, 1538-3636 (Electronic) 0003-990X (Linking)

[46] Kegeles, L. S., Abi-Dargham, A., Frankle, W. G., Gil, R., Cooper, T. B., Slifstein, M., Hwang, D. R., Huang, Y., Haber, S. N.& Laruelle, M. (2010): Increased synaptic dopamine function in associative regions of the striatum in schizophrenia. *Arch Gen Psychiatry*, Vol. 67, No. 3,pp.231-239, 1538-3636 (Electronic) 0003-990X (Linking)

[47] Howes, O. D., Montgomery, A. J., Asselin, M. C., Murray, R. M., Valli, I., Tabraham, P., Bramon-Bosch, E., Valmaggia, L., Johns, L., Broome, M., McGuire, P. K.& Grasby, P. M. (2009): Elevated striatal dopamine function linked to prodromal signs of schizophrenia. *Arch Gen Psychiatry*, Vol. 66, No. 1,pp.13-20, 1538-3636 (Electronic) 0003-990X (Linking)

[48] Costafreda, S. G., Fu, C. H., Picchioni, M., Kane, F., McDonald, C., Prata, D. P., Kalidindi, S., Walshe, M., Curtis, V., Bramon, E., Kravariti, E., Marshall, N., Toulopoulou, T., Barker, G. J., David, A. S., Brammer, M. J., Murray, R. M.& McGuire, P. K. (2009): Increased inferior frontal activation during word generation: a marker of genetic risk for schizophrenia but not bipolar disorder? *Hum Brain Mapp*, Vol. 30, No. 10,pp.3287-3298, 1097-0193 (Electronic) 1065-9471 (Linking)

[49] Haber, S. N. (2003): The primate basal ganglia: parallel and integrative networks. *J Chem Neuroanat*, Vol. 26, No. 4,pp.317-330, 0891-0618 (Print) 0891-0618 (Linking)

[50] Middleton, F. A.& Strick, P. L. (2000): Basal ganglia and cerebellar loops: motor and cognitive circuits. *Brain Res Brain Res Rev*, Vol. 31, No. 2-3,pp.236-250,

[51] Simpson, E. H., Kellendonk, C., Ward, R. D., Richards, V., Lipatova, O., Fairhurst, S., Kandel, E. R.& Balsam, P. D. (2011): Pharmacologic rescue of motivational deficit in an animal model of the negative symptoms of schizophrenia. *Biol Psychiatry*, Vol. 69, No. 10,pp.928-935, 1873-2402 (Electronic) 0006-3223 (Linking)

Chapter 6

Sexual Dimorphism in Human Teeth from Dental Morphology and Dimensions: A Dental Anthropology Viewpoint

Freddy Moreno-Gómez

Additional information is available at the end of the chapter

http://dx.doi.org/10.5772/55881

1. Introduction

Based on the referenced literature and from a holistic and integrating viewpoint, dental anthropology is seen as an interdisciplinary field that integrates knowledge of anthropology, dentistry, biology, paleontology and paleopathology in order to study all the information provided by the human dentition, such as anatomical, developmental, pathological, cultural and therapeutic variations in consideration of the conditions of life, culture, food and adaptation processes of the past and present human populations, through morphology, size, disease and modifications of teeth [1,2].

Basically, dental anthropology is concerned with the study of morphological variation (dental morphological features) and metrics of the dentition of human populations over time (prehistoric and modern) and space (ethnic influences) and their relation with the processes of adaptation and dietary changes that led to the evolution of the dental system and the human race [3]. This is possible because the enamel is the hardest tissue of the human body and has a high capacity to preserve itself even in extreme conditions of pH, moisture, salinity and high temperatures, which is recognized in the archaeological taphonomic field as resistance, that dental morphology is expressed to be genetically unique and unrepeatable in each tooth [4], and the tooth structure (metric and morphological) formed histoembryologically does not change or remodel itself as with the bone, excluding mechanical wear or attrition and accumulation of secondary dentine [1], and teeth, in many cases have become the only element to be able *per se* to provide biological and cultural information of an individual or a human population, which is possible due to: 1. High heritability and strong genetic control of dental morphology; 2. Little environmental influence; 3. Correspondence between the dental characteristics and geographical distribution; 4. Are easy to observe and record; 5. Permit to compare past with present populations; 6. Have the ability to reflect the dietary habits of an individual and how they process food; 7. Reveal the conditions of health, age, sex, habits and functional occupational habits; and 8. Make evident technological and cultural development of a population [5-9].

Similarly, in the forensic context, the dentition is the accurate way to identify individuals whose death makes it difficult to distinguish by other processes (visual recognition, fingerprints, documents and clothing), which contributes to the reconstruction of individual and general osteo-biography (odonto-biography in the case of the teeth) (10]. That is, in anthropological and forensic contexts initially it is established general biology that links the individual as a member of a population with a specific gender, a certain age, ethnic patterns and a series of detailed physical characteristics including height and body proportions, commonly referred to as the basic quartet of identification. However, the diagnosis of sex is successful in 100% of the cases when the skeleton is complete and in good condition, when the individual is an adult and when the intra-group morphometric variability of the population, which the specimen belongs, is known. If only is available the skull, in an unknown population context or if the individual is immature, the degree of objectivity can range from 80 to 90%, taking into account that the age group between 15-18 years is the age limit to from which the sexual estimate more accurately appreciated [11].

2. Sexual dimorphism in human teeth

Human populations vary according to their phylogenetic origins as macro and micro-evolutionary patterns, ethnic, sexual characteristics (gender) and ontogenetically by age and also there are individual variations of each human being as a member of a species. That is why in the anthropological context, the population analysis is done through levels or scales ranging from general to particular and individual from the individual, the intra-group and inter-group, which is recognized as basic identification quatrain, which includes age, ethnic pattern, height and gender. The latter seeks from sexual variations on the shape and size of individuals, whether an individual is female, male or allophys, in which case it is not possible to determine either gender. This set of variations in ethnic and phylogenetic origin is known as sexual dimorphism. Contemporary humans are dimorphic, but less so than other hominids, with a body sexual dimorphism index of only 4 to 7%. However, taking into account the morphological features of post-cranial skeleton increases from 8 to 20% and that from the teeth increases 8 to 9%, mainly in the canine teeth, which are considered the most dimorphic teeth of living current human [6].

To determine the sex in the anthropological context from skeletal remains, there are different methods to analyze the metrical features or dimensions of the skull, which is known as craniometry, the morphological features or shape of the skull, including the glabella, the supra-orbital ridge, the nuchal crest, mastoid process and the chin, the bones of the skeleton as the jaw, hip, sacrum, scapula, clavicle, sternum, humerus and femur mainly, and metric and morphological features of teeth (10]. Through analysis of teeth, it is possible to study the sexual dimorphism of an individual from the patterns of dental development and eruption, the expression of a protein known as amelogenin, dental morphology and dental dimensions.

3. Dental morphology

The odontoscopy or study of dental morphology, from the concept given by dental anthropology seeks to observe, record, analyze and understand the behavior of the expression (frequency and variability) of coronal and root morphology of human teeth. Overall, the teeth morphology is formed by a number of features that have been called dental crown and root traits, which constitute the enamel phenotypic forms expressed and regulated by the genome of an individual and a population during odontogenesis. These can be positive structures (tubercular and radicular) or negative (pit form and intertubercular) that have the potential to be present or not in a specific location (frequency) in different ways (variability) in one or more members of a population group [2,13-14]. Thus, the study of dental morphology integrates different disciplines such as physical anthropology, biology, dentistry, paleontology and paleopathology, with the aim of generating markers from the teeth of both primitive and the modern human being, characterizing the taxonomy of the human species within the anthropological context and following a crucial role in the processes of identification for forensic purposes, since the teeth and dental morphology is a highly heritable characteristic, that have the potential to establish classifications, allow comparison of the primitive with the modern restoration materials, are stable in time and have a fairly high state of preservation compared to the bone material [15].

3.1. Non-metric dental traits

The dental morphological or non-metric characters, are also called discrete, discontinuous, quasi-continuous or epigenetic traits [7] and they are observed, recorded and analyzed with scientific evidence of high taxonomic value, frequency, variability, bilaterallity, sexual dimorphism and correspondence between features, conditions that allow them to be used in the estimation of biological relationships among populations by comparative analysis of human past and present groups, to try to clarify the historical, cultural and biological macro-and micro-evolution, leading to the understanding of displacement, migration paths and contacts that led to the settlement and ethnic variation of humanity. All existing studies indicate that dental morphological traits have a strong genetic component if one takes into account their occurrence or frequency and the expression or gradation [6].

The analysis of dental morphology, parallel to the genetic observation is based on the frequency and variability of non-metric dental traits through the phenetic method (the phenome is the physical expression of the genome) applied especially for the comparison of population frequencies i.e. a dental morphological feature is the representation of an elementary and indivisible taxonomic trait known as phen (phenetic variation unit) which, as a feature discrete dichotomy is expressed by the presence - absence initially described by A. Hrdlicka in 1920 after observing the characteristic shovel-shaped incisors concluding that when a feature was present it took different forms, ranging from minimal forms of expression to maximum levels. It is for this reason that for the population phenetic analysis is used stable dental crown traits and high genetic component, which determine the grade of variations or degrees of expression. For this purpose, must be selected samples of at least

100 individuals per population phenotypically different from the standpoint of inter-group. In this way are found the more effective degrees of a taxonomic trait selected in order to obtain inter-group markers in a specific population [6].

Until present, there are over 100 dental crown traits and root that have been recognized in the human dentition, but in most worldwide research are used no more than 17 features, mainly those located in the crown of incisors and molars of both dentitions. The observation of these features is done through different methods reported in the literature, excelling ASUDAS method (16] developed since 1940 by A. Dahlberg from standard dental plates and transferred in 1981 to C. G. Turner II at Department of Anthropology of the Arizona State University, hence its name.

However, different authors have developed their own monitoring systems for different morphological features, both for deciduous and permanent teeth, such as methods of K. Hanihara [17], A. Zoubov [15], K. Alt [13], P. Sciulli [18], and F. Grine [19], among others. These systems generally allow observation beyond the dichotomy of presence/absence and promote inter-observer reproducibility to generate data that represent physical minimum and maximum expression of a trait and varying degrees of expression between these two reference points.

To make the correct observation and grading of dental morphological traits are used models of plaster casts of dental impressions in polymeric materials with high dimensional stability from individuals of a particular population. The observer, previously calibrated, learn to handle morphological systems used on plaster models with the aid of a stereomicroscope and a fine tip dental explorer. Generally, from the statistical point of view, estimating the degree of agreement takes into account the criteria of inter-observer (observer vs. gold standard) and intra-observer (observer vs. observer) denoted by C. R. Nichol and C. G. Turner [20]. To define the dental morphological features, mainly expressed in the crown of the tooth will be grouped by the type of teeth (incisors, canines, premolars and molars), with the aim of demonstrating their sexual dimorphism expression (frequency), variability (gradation) bilateral symmetry, correspondence between biological traits and population distances. To name each tooth is possible to use two types of nomenclature, FDI (World Dental Federation) and anthropologic nomenclature. In the FDI nomenclature, 32 permanent and 20 deciduous teeth are divided into hemi-arches and each hemi-arch is named with a number, 1 for the upper right hemi-arch, 2 for the upper left hemi-arch, 3 for lower left hemi-arch and 4 for the lower right hemi-arch. The first digit representing a tooth indicates the hemi-arch where the tooth is located. In the case of primary teeth quadrants are represented by the numbers 5 to the upper right hemi-arch, 6 for the upper left hemi-arch, 7 for the lower left hemi-arch and 8 for the lower right hemi-arch. For example, for tooth number 11, which is a central incisor, the first 1corresponds to upper right hemi-arch, the second 1 corresponds to the position from mesial to distal, so it is a permanent right maxillary central incisor. In the case of anthropological nomenclature, the teeth are represented by an alphanumeric code where the dental arch is represented by the "U" for upper arch and "L" for the lower arch, the tooth class is named with the same initial, "I" for incisors, "C" for canines, "P" for premolars and "M" for molar, and if in a class of two types of teeth will be numbered according to position. This corresponds to the UI2 maxillary lateral incisor. For the primary dentition is used the same code but are in lowercase alphabetic characters. Since in the anthropological context of bilateral symmetry classes and types of teeth are fully established, there is no discrimination if left or right.

3.1.1. Incisors

In human primary and permanent dentition, there are two types of incisors, upper central incisors UI1 (11 and 21) and LI1 lower (31 and 41), located on either side of the midline, and the upper lateral incisors UI2 (12 and 22) and LI2 lower (32 and 42), which are available immediately distal of the central incisors. These, along with the canines are the group of anterior teeth, whose most basic functions are the arrest (along with the lips), the incision and the partition of food into smaller pieces so they can be chewed by the posterior teeth. They also have an important role in functions of the human being as passive participation in phonation and a complex social component such as an active part of the aesthetic facial [21-23]. Both in primary and permanent incisors there have been reported several dental crown traits like winging (rotation of one or both maxillary central incisors with respect to the midline), crowding (crowding of the incisors), shovel-shaped (development of the mesial and distal marginal ridges), double shovel-shaped (relative development of the buccal marginal ridge setting up a sort of pit vestibular), dental tubercle (crest or tubercle which appears in the region of the cingulum on the lingual surface), interruption groove (across the cingulate sulcus to reach the enamel-cement, often continues into the root), curvature of the labial surface (convex in the middle third of the labial surface of the crown surface viewed from the incisal) and vestibular contour (contour shape of the incisors in relation to the mesial and distal marginal ridges, the incisal and cervical margins) [24-27].

This chapter will be described the shovel-shape as a feature of great forensic and anthropology interest.

- Shovel-shaped

It consists of the marked development of the mesial and distal marginal ridges and palatal configuration of the deep pit in a triangle. Is seen mainly in the upper central incisors, although the feature can be expressed in the upper lateral and less frequently in both lower incisors, however, in the population analysis only the central incisor is used as inter-group marker to be a polar stable tooth, according to the statement of the theory of morphogenetic fields of P. Butler [6]. The observation method was proposed by A. Hrdlicka in 1920, the plate was developed by A. Dahlberg in 1956 and the current classification was made by G. Scott in 1970. The reference plate in the ASU system is UI1 ASUDAS shovel. The blade shape is observed in the lingual surface of central incisors and upper and lower side, formed by the palate or lingual fossa and mesial and distal marginal ridges [16]. The dichotomous expression (presence/absence) describe from a flat palatal surface to a marked development of the marginal ridges. For the taxonomic analysis are only taken into account the marginal ridges and not the depth of the concavity since the latter is quite independent and has negative correlation with the development of the ridges. However, some authors take into account the depth of the pit palate and indicate that there is shovel-shaped from 0.5 mm in depth, if less does not express the trait [28].

The worldwide variation of this marker in the central incisors ranges from 5% in Europe to 100% in Mongoloid origin populations. Since the time of early African hominids it has been showed the development of shovel-shaped incisors. In Asia this trait is clearly expressed since the early hominids. According to paleontological information, exists a geographical boundary between the West, with low frequencies of shovel incisors, and the east with high frequencies of this trait [6], which is an effective boundary between the European and Mongoloid populations (Asian and American) [15].

K. Hanihara [17] developed the Mongoloid dental complex from five dental morphological traits (including shovel-shaped upper central incisors) that had a high frequency and distribution of which were quite useful in analyzing the affinities between different populations. Thus, for this trait expression there are differences between Negroid, Caucasian-American and Mongoloid origin population groups. In particular, significantly higher frequencies are shown by Japanese, Pimas and Eskimos, and slightly less in Ainu. T. Hanihara [28] found a prevalence of 9.2% in Japanese, 33.3% in blacks and 27.7% in white Americans, while C. G. Turner in (1984) observed this trait in 98.8% of sinodontes, in 99.8% of the South American aborigins and in 29.4% of northeastern Europeans. The same C. G. Turner II [29-31] related the results of the frequencies of some morphological traits of populations of Asia, Oceania a Polynesia and Hispanic American populations, and in this way he showed that the Americas were populated via the Bering Strait. Similarly, the geographic distribution of traits according to different human groups that make up the dental complex East Asian Mongoloid allowed Sinodonte subdivide the pattern in the north, characterized by the addition and enhancement of some features (like the shovel incisors), and the pattern Sundadonte south, typified by the retention of an ancestral condition and simplification of certain features within the protruding low frequency of shovel-shaped. Would be those who crossed the Bering Sinodontos some 14,000 years ago who populated the Americas in three consecutive waves, being the east of Lake Baikal the last home of the indigenous peoples of North and South America. Therefore, all pre-Columbian indigenous groups are part of the pattern Sinodonto at the Mongoloid dental complex. For this reason, the shovel shaped central incisors are present in almost 100% of pre-Hispanic and American Indian populations in modern American populations as evidence of the process of miscegenation [24-27].

3.1.2. Canines

Anatomically, the canines have bulkier root in the palatal-lingual direction and longer than other teeth, this allows a strong anchoring in the alveolar bone with abundant and dense compact bone and confers high resilience to the forces generated during the chewing cycle during which dampen excessive horizontal and deleterious forces are generated during lateral movements to protect the back teeth, an action that depends equally from its high capacity to nociceptive sensory stimuli during the action of mastication muscles. Basically, this protection is mediated by the occlusal relationship between the canines, which, upon the lateral movement of the lower canines jaw slide over the top, a function described in the literature as "canine function" or "canine key," to produce disoclussion of posterior teeth. Hence, the canines are considered "milestones" or "signposts" of dental occlusion. These consist of two maxillary and two mandibular teeth localized each one in a hemiarch between the incisors and premolars group. The upper canine crown UC (13 and 23) presents the labial surface in a diamond shape, with the incisal edge acute (formed by the mesial and distal cusp slopes that meet at a cusp vertex) and rounded in the cervical region. The palatal surface has a central crest elevation or extension from the cingulum to the cusp apex, and two marginal ridges, mesial and distal, which constitute the central ridge with two mesial and distal palatal fossae respectively. The lower canines LC [33, 43] have a longer narrower crown, and lower bulge than the upper canines. From the buccal view, mesial contour is relatively straight while the concave distal cementoenamel junction, but convex in the distal cusp slope. On the lingual surface mesial and distal pits are less noticeable than in the upper, and the cingulum is more blunt than the upper canine and the mesial and distal halves of the crown are more symmetrical. Permanent canines are the only teeth in its class in both the maxilla and mandible, where they are located at the four corners of the dental arches between the lateral incisors and first premolars, what constitutes an important support of the facial muscles. Phylogenetically, morphology and dimensions have been associated with capture functions, excavation, cutting, boring, defense, attack, sexual dimorphism and social power [21-23].

In the case of the canines very few studies have been conducted. P. Butler in 1939 suggested that the morphology and size of the premolars are controlled by the canines ("caninization" of the first premolars) and molars ("molarization" of the second premolars) during tooth morphogenesis, while A. Dahlberg in 1945 held that the premolars had a morphogenetic field independent and exclusive to them. In short, none of the two theories have been proven due to the exclusion of the premolars of anthropological and genetic research (largely due to ignorance of evolutionary and embryological behavior of these teeth), being relegated from the global dental morphological classifications (dental complex) and limited their study to the description of the meso-distal and bucco-palatal or bucco-lingual dimensions [32].

Worldwide research on this topic has covered many of the current populations and a number of past populations, focusing mainly on the description of the frequency and variability of dental morphological features located in incisors and molars, leaving aside the morphology of canines and premolars. However, the descriptive and quantitative analysis of the morphology of the canines has allowed hominids to be taxonomically classified, so that has contributed to the estimate of the evolutionary origin of the genus *Homo* and understanding the geographical distribution of past and modern human groups. In primates, the reduction in canine size and degree of sexual dimorphism is related to the size of the crown and the simplification of the morphology, which received direct selective pressure from the acquisition of the erect position, the bipedalism, reduced facial prognathism, reducing the size of the dental arches and microdontia generalized morphological conditions specific to humans [33-35].

In the temporary and permanent canines, according to reports in the literature, it is possible to study various dental crown traits such as shovel-shaped (relative development of the mesial and distal marginal ridges of the lingual surface), double shovel (relative development the mesial and distal marginal ridges on the labial surface), labial convexity (convexity degree of vestibular), slot interrupt (through the cingulate sulcus of the upper canines up to the cement-enamel junction), dental tubercle (crest, tubercle or peak that appears in the cingulate region of the lingual surface), canine mesial ridge (mesial crest variation), distal accessory ridge (small accessory crest that appears on the distal-incisal) central peak (central area shown in palate), palatal fossae (two graves, mesial and distal, which appear in the palatal surface of the upper canines) and lingual fossae (two graves, mesial and distal, which appear on the lingual surface of the lower canines) (36]. The canine mesial ridge and the distal accessory ridge are population dental traits important within anthropological and forensic contexts.

- Mesial canine ridge

The expression is observed in the variation of the mesial crest of the upper canines. The canine mesial ridge, the protostylid or "Bushman canine" was described by Morris in a population of Bushmen in South Africa [37]. The recording of this feature is done by ASU Bushman Canine plate [16], which describes such a way that the mesiolingual edge of the upper canine, similar in size to distolingual, can overcome and form a fold distal approximately 2/3 below the incisal surface, due to its junction with the dental tubercle.

- Distal accessory ridge

It is observed as the presence and expression of a small accessory crest that appears on the distal-incisal region of upper and lower canines. The record of this trait was performed by UC DAR ASU board. This has been one of the most worldwide studied morphological crown dental traits of canines [16]

3.1.3. Premolars

In the case of the premolars are very few studies conducted. P. Butler in 1939 suggested that the morphology and size of the premolars are controlled by the canines ("caninization" of the first premolars) and molars ("molarization" of the second premolars) during tooth morphogenesis, while A. A. Dahlberg in 1945 held that the premolars have a morphogenetic field independent and exclusive to them. In short, none of the two theories have been proven to the exclusion of the premolars of anthropological and genetic research (largely due to ignorance of evolutionary and embryological behavior of these teeth), being relegated from the global dental morphological classifications (dental complex) and limited their study to the description of the meso-distal an bucco-palatal or bucco-lingual dimensions [38].

The premolars consist of four maxillary and four mandibular teeth located in pairs on each hemiarch between the canines and first molars. The higher UP1 (14 and 24) and UP2 (15 and 25) have two cusps of similar size and usually two roots, especially the first premolar. The occlusal surface has an oval contour characterized by well-defined grooves directed from mesial to distal. The lower LP1 (34 and 44) and LP2 (35 and 45) are uniradicular, and have three cusps (second premolar) that form a rounded occlusal contour with a groove, which is often interrupted. Broadly speaking, the premolars are a transition from the canine (buccal cusp high and pointed cone), which increase the occlusal contour from the first to the second, i.e. "molarization" thanks to the development of prominent marginal ridges and increased height of the palate or lingual cusp [21-23].

In the literature have been reported and described as 12 dental crown traits, such as the mesial accessory ridge (small ridge located toward mesial of accessory sagittal grooves), distal accessory ridge (homologous mesial accessory crest, but is located towards distal of the buccal cusp of the maxillary premolars), mesial interstitial tubercle (tuber apex or blunt cusp mesial region between the buccal and palatal cusps of the premolars), distal interstitial tubercle (or Terra, cusp or tubercle apex blunt cusp between the distal buccal and palatal cusps of the premolars), tricuspid bicuspid (developed disto-lingual cusp is smaller and closer to the palatal cusp), hypostyle (small cusp with vertex set which usually appears between the buccal cusp and disto-lingual cusp), vestibular sulcus (odontogliphyc feature that is the distal groove projecting from the distal pit to buccal), central ridge (or ridge of enamel bridge that connects the buccal cusp with meso-lingual cusp), meso-lingual sulcus (odontogliphyc trait that describes the path that part of the hole and crosses the mesial marginal ridge towards the same side of meso-lingual), disto-lingual groove (odontogliphyc trait that corresponds to groove originate from the distal marginal ridge and crosses the same side of the distal-lingual direction), lingual cusp number (number of cusps that can occur in the region of first premolar lingual) and groove pattern (configuration of the grooves and the contact pattern of the cusps of the occlusal surface of the lower premolars) [39].

The frequencies reported by G. Giron et al [39] show the trend of the first premolar to have a low frequency of mesial accessory crest and a moderate expression of distal accessory ridge, two cusps with constant presence, absence of buccal grooves and lower frequencies of interstitial tubercle mesial and distal, while the second premolars often show high expression of the mesial and distal accessory ridges, and the interstitial tubercles mesial and distal (although the expression of this trait in the first premolars in the latter is greater); likewise always have two cusps and no developmental grooves vestibular are expressed. In the case of the lower premolars, the first is characterized by no vestibular developmental grooves, only one lingual cusp present, have a high central peak expression, mesiolingual groove and a U-groove pattern, in contrast to the configuration of the occlusal morphology of lower second premolars which is very different, given the low expression of meso-and disto lingual groove, the absence of central ridge and vestibular groove, the high frequency of a single lingual cusp and groove U pattern.

3.1.4. Molars

The molar teeth consist of four maxillary and four mandibular teeth located in pairs on each hemiarch distal of the canines. The UM2 second molars (55 and 65) and lower LM2 (75 and

85) are totally different from the first molars UM1 (54 and 64) and LM1 (74 and 84) and have a shape and morphological features very similar to the first permanent molars. The first molars are not taken into account because, although their morphology is very variable, they are more like a premolar than a molar. Permanent molars are six maxillar and six mandibular, which are located distal to the second premolars. UM1 first upper (16 and 26) and lower molars LM1 (36 and 46) and UM2 upper (17 and 27) and lower LM2 second molars (37 and 47) at first glance are very similar, but under analysis of dental anthropology, they have significant differences in the expression of dental crown traits, which is why the same correspondence between one and other tooth will permit to understand the genetic and environmental influences, both by their frequency the expression. UM3 third molars (18 and 28) and LM3 (38 and 48) are not taken into account for the study of dental morphology since this tooth has a strong evolutionary trend toward the disappearance, which is evident given the high frequency of agenesis and atypical forms [21-23].

In the molars the traits that have been more frequently studied are Carabelli trait (pit or cusp in the meso-lingual cusp of the upper molars), hypoconid reduction (downsizing disto-lingual cusp of the upper molars), metaconulo (small cusp between disto-buccal cusp and disto-palatal maxillary molars) groove pattern (contact configuration of the cusps of the molars), number of cusps, elbow crease (the meso-lingual cusp is directed toward the central fossa in lower molars), protostylid (pit or buccal cusp on the buccal developmental groove of the mandibular molars), cusp 6 (cusp between the disto-buccal cusp and disto-lingual surfaces of lower molars) and cusp 7 (cusp between the meso-lingual cusp and disto-lingual surfaces of lower molars) [24-27].

The features to be the focus of the discussion in this chapter are the most studied in worldwide populations, as in the case of the cusp of Carabelli, protostylid and groove pattern.

- Carabelli trait

It is located on the palatal surface of the apex of the mesopalatal cusp of second primary molar and the first and second upper permanent molars. The variability of expression ranges from a small pit, through a groove in a "V" or "Y" up to the formation of a cusp. The first observation scale was developed by A. Dahlberg in 1956. One of the methods of measurement in the primary dentition was designed by F. Grine [19], while for permanent teeth are usually used the ASUDAS method developed by C. G. Turner [16].

Carabelli trait is considered worldwide as a Caucasoid trait. T. Hanihara [28] found low frequencies of this trait in Japanese and higher in black and white Americans, finding that this trait distinguishes Caucasoid populations of Asian and that in the latter predominate the groove and pit forms, whereas C. G. Turner [29] found significant expressions in sinodontes, South American indigenous and northeastern Europeans.

In modern American populations, N. Aragon et al [27] in a sample of an indigenous population in Colombia found that in both dentitions dominated groove and pit forms (grades 1 and 2 in deciduous, grades 1 to 4 in permanent teeth) than cusp form (degree 3 and 4 in deciduous, grades 5 to 7 in permanent). However, and according to the expression dichotomy, although the cusp of Carabelli is considered to be present in the sample should not be associated as a product of mixing of Caucasoid origin, since the intermediate grades pit expression is considered present and is characteristic of American Indian populations. J. Rocha et al [26] in a population of Afro-Colombians in Colombia found significant frequencies of cusp expression, which is characteristic of populations of African origin and that according to A. Zoubov [15], conform southern Caucasoid dental or western equatorial complex. In a mixed population of Colombia, S. Moreno et al [24] reported the higher frequencies in grades 0, 1 and 2 with a higher prevalence of grade 1 (fovea present). L. Aguirre et al [25] indicated that the cusp of Carabelli is not sexually dimorphic, it is expressed predominantly bilaterally and furrow and grave forms of tubercle and cusp forms, both as permanent dentition, which indicates that there is ambivalence in discrimination population for this trait. The correlation of the prevalence between both dentitions indicates a strong genetic control for the expression of it.

- Protostylid

This paramolar cusp is antagonist to Carabelli cusp that varies from a groove to a free apex cusp on the vestibular surface of the meso-vestibular cusp. Also is often expressed as a fovea or pit on the buccal developmental groove called Point P or vestibular foramen caecum. A. Dahlberg developed the reference plate in 1956 [6], but at present the method to observe it in permanent molars is ASUDAS [16].

A. Zoubov [15] defines americanoide protostylid as a feature due to the low frequency of expression in the populations of Europe, Africa and Asia the peculiarity of the high prevalence of point P or foramen caecum American populations. K. Hanihara [40,41] indicated that the expression of protostylid cusp is rarely present in different populations, occurring rarely in modern human groups, most Asians, which allow to differentiate the dental complex of Caucasoid and Mongoloid Negroid. In primary teeth is commonly observed pit expression and some degree of mild elevations. N. Aragon et al [27] found this feature absent from the sample in the case of primary dentition and present with groove expression in the permanent dentition in an indigenous Colombian sample. The interesting thing about this feature is the high frequency of grade 1 (pit or foramen caecum) in primary teeth, and that although in permanent teeth is often the development of the distal row from vestibular sulcus, is a preserved expression of the form pit. J. Rocha et al [26] described the protostylid as absent in the sample of African descent, but they highlight the high frequency of grade 1 which again suggests the possibility of interbreeding with indigenous peoples, in the same way as S. Moreno et al [24] in their study in a mixed population of Caucasoid Colombians reported high frequency of grade 1. L. Aguirre et al [25] in their study observed that the protostylid reflects that the population studied has a significant retention of American Indian dental complex, as evidenced by the high frequency of grade 1, explained as a pit on the buccal developmental groove that separates meso and disto-buccal cusps. These authors state that in modern American populations the protostylid pit form predominates in both deciduous and permanent dentition.

- Groove pattern

The groove pattern of the second temporary molars and first permanent molars describes the configuration of the contact of the cusps and the number of them. The classic pattern is Y or "Driopitecino" originating in the past Asian populations, and + X or "cruciform" are considered as reductions frequently observed in Caucasoid groups [6]. N. Aragon et al [27] report that the behavior of the number of cusps and groove pattern, present for the case of deciduous dentition Y6 and Y7 predominantly configuration, where the groove pattern and has a strong genetic control kept from past Asian populations that inhabited the Americas through Beringia from which derive the pre-hispanic Amerindian and present populations. In their study of African descent, J. Rocha et al [26] found that the behavior of the groove pattern and number of cusps shows the predominance of +5 and +6 configuration, shown as a reduction driopitecino pattern characteristic of non-Mongoloid populations. The frequencies of the configurations X6 and Y5 suggest some genetic influence product of miscegenation of Caucasian and indigenous groups. L. Aguirre et al [25] reported that expression of the grooves intercuspal contact was given by the Y pattern for the second temporary molars and + pattern for the first permanent molars, indicating that it may be because the primary dentition has a strong genetic control and has therefore retained the original Driopitecino pattern of ancestral Asian populations. In the case of the first permanent molars, one can assume that the miscegenation processes mark a trend toward + pattern, which is characteristic of Caucasian populations.

3.2. Sexual dimorphism of dental morphological traits

3.2.1. Incisors

Regarding the incisor teeth, in the literature can be found a general consensus of the absence of sexual dimorphism in the shovel form, taken into account in this chapter that this is one of the most studied dental traits for its importance in the discrimination populations according to the dental complex. However, in the dental literature, there are several reports describing morphological differences according to sex of individuals and has great clinical importance in the area of aesthetic and cosmetic dentistry for diagnostic procedures of smile design [42]. Thus, the proximal contours, dental angle, incisal edge and the emergence profile are important for the teeth in harmony with the shape of the face [43-44].

Within the body outline the face has an aesthetic requirement that is extremely important as the aesthetic composition of the human as psycho-socio-cultural being, and teeth are part of the integral and harmonious appearance of the morpho-functional composition, including within the aesthetic-affective manifestations recognized as smiling, laughing, kissing and oral-facial gestures being teeth beyond the biological part of the smile. Their disposition in the arches are in compliance with the support function of the soft tissues, influencing the position taken by the facial muscles, which contribute to the determination of facial traits that are involved in the character and personality. For this reason, the face and facial expression are influenced by genetic inheritance and environmental factors, within which are the rounded, square or triangular shape of upper central incisors [45-47].

The analysis of these and other structures that make up the stomatognathic system of human groups, constitutes a fundamental starting point for micro-and macro-historical processes and reconstruction of the ethno-demographic origin of the current populations, for biological, functional and aesthetic dental diagnosis prognosis and treatment plans, and for forensic identification methods using facial reconstruction techniques.

Williams in 1914 -cited by L. Ibrahimagi et al [48]- postulated that the inverted form of the upper central incisors is related to the shape of the face, which is applicable in dental settings for harmonization of aesthetic oral rehabilitation procedures, anthropological (morphological grounds for facial reconstruction procedure) and forensic (individualization during the identification process). Frush and Fisher -cited by M. Waliszewski [49]- proposed the concept of "genetic tooth aesthetic form of the patient", which indicate that the shape of the teeth due to factors such as sex, age and personality of the patient, which coined the term dentogenic to name the relationship between these variables. But there is no consensus in the various literature reports. Wright and Brodbelt, -cited by L. Ibrahimagi et al [48]- reported that the shape of the upper central incisors and the shape of the face corresponds to a situation that had already expressed by the same Ibrahimagi et al [48] in disagreement with the theory of Williams mainly because the mix of ethnic groups in the population and the infinite possibilities of combining forms of differently shaped face and the upper central incisors shape had selectively affected the genetic correlation between these two variables. S. Berksun et al [50] and S. Wolfart et al [51] reported that it is possible to define the correlation of the shape of the face and shape of the teeth due to ethnic ambiguity of worldwide reports. Thus, D. Acosta et al [52] conducted a study in Caucasian population where correlated features as facial contour with the shape of the contour of the upper central incisors, finding that an oval facial shape corresponds to the oval shaped upper central incisors, which does not occurs with square and triangular shapes. Likewise, although there is significant sexual dimorphism in the shape or contour of the face or the shape of the contour of the upper central incisors, the authors conclude that women had more prevalent oval and round shapes, while than in men predominate oval and square shapes.

3.2.2. Canines

The study of canine morphology has been used to understand the evolution of sexual dimorphism in the socio-ecological and phylogenetic development of primates. Sexual dimorphism is defined as an intra-specific difference between men and women, which can be studied from the somatotype of the individual, the size and dental morphology, and correlated with intra-sexual patterns of competition [53,54]. Ontogenetic mechanisms exist that cause morphological differences between males and females during primate evolution. The ontogenetic changes in these processes lead to the existence of sexual dimorphism associated with the size and evolutionary response to various factors including territoriality, competition and the distribution of resources [55].

Despite the changes in the size of the canines during hominid evolutionary line between male and female individuals, morphology has not suffered sexual dimorphism given its high intra-species preservation, related primarily to the canine is the one of a kind and has its own highly conserved morphogenetic field, which is also supported by the bilateral symmetry of dental morphological traits [35].

P. Butler since 1937-cited by van Reenen et al [56] - from his studies in Cenozoic mammals under the concepts of Huxley and De Beer, formulated the theory of morphogenetic fields in which the ectomesenchyme that migrates within the first arch is programmed to form a single tooth family that later modify its form by the action of external factors. In 1945, A. Dahlberg -cited by van Reenen et al [56] - adapts the concept of morphogenetic fields in the human dentition and represents the existence of four rather than three dental fields, and introduces the premolar class as a field. While it should be noted that the deciduous and permanent molars have similar morphological characteristics that allow them to be linked to the same morphogenetic field, in man and in most mammals premolars differ markedly from their predecessors, the molars, and this is why premolars could be considered as potential molars deviated the field development by the molar (molarization) and were influenced by proximity to canine field (caninizaion). Later, G. C. Scott and C. G. Turner [5] suggested that gradients expressed in the morphogenetic field theory and the model proposed by Osborn clones theory in 1978, in which, as ectomesenchyme migrates into the first arc, and is differentiated into three clones, incisor, canine and molar, have scientific evidence and do not exclude each other.

Today, advances in molecular biology have allowed to mark the factors that control the morphogenesis of teeth from epithelial-mesenchymal relationships, in fact, the morphogenetic field corresponds to a specific place where a number of factors and proteins development are expressed and inhibited in the formation of a specific tooth, so bilateral symmetry and the absence of sexual dimorphism in the expression of dental morphological features of the canine teeth is associated with temporary and permanent mainly to the canines are the teeth of the morphogenetic field gradient, and as the central incisors and first molars for their respective fields, they are in the teeth with higher degree of conservation according to gene expression and lower influence of the environment from the viewpoint of macro-evolution.

3.2.3. *Premolars*

In the case of the premolars, the shape of its contour and dimensions have been extensively studied as a tool for building the phylogeny of hominids from small samples of Australopithecines, Pliocene hominids, and Homo of low and medium Pleistocene [57], because from the standpoint of dental anthropology, the evolutionary value of morphology and dental odontometry is based on the strong genetic control of frequency and variability, which allows to establish direct links between the anatomical structure of the teeth, including premolars, and relationship between populations. However, in the literature are few studies on morphology of premolars and there have not been studied all the morphological features or have used different methodologies, based on the likelihood that human groups that present a similar dental morphology and dimensions can be interrelated, in fact, the shape and dimensions exhibited by a tooth-set the similarity or dissimilarity of morphological variation and genetic metric of a common ethnic trunk [58]. This will make it possible to infer macro-evolutionary processes that have demarcated the settlement, in this case a specific region such as the southwestern Colombia.

Based on the frequency and variability of morphological features obtained in this study, graphically presents the morphology of the occlusal surface of a sample of mixed Caucasoid traits of the first and second upper and lower premolars. To demonstrate the behavior of the expression of the morphology of the premolars has important clinical implications (in the dental context) whenever the functional morphology plays a role in inter-occlusal relationships during the various functions of the stomatognathic system [21-23] and ethnic (in the anthropological and forensic contexts), because there is ample evidence in the literature analysis tooth morphology contributes to the establishment of the basic identification quatrain (osteography or odontography) specifically in the estimation of the age, sex and ethnic pattern [59,60].

Regarding the theory of morphogenetic fields made by P. Butler, in which the morphology of the deciduous and permanent teeth due to a progressive gradation from the incisors to the molars, premolars can be considered as potential deviated molars from field development influenced by the molar (molarization) and that, as stated previously, the field were influenced canine (caninization), so that the conformation of the occlusal table from the development of cusps and the expansion of meso-distal and bucco palatal or bucco lingual diameters. However, the deciduous molars have the same characteristics of permanent molars (for which they are associated with a single morphogenetic field), while the premolars differ markedly from their predecessors, the molars. This occurs in most mammals, including man, so A. Dahlberg adapted the concept of morphogenetic fields in the human dentition and justified the existence of four fields, where the premolars molars have their own field. This theory was supported by Scott and Turner, indicating that the shape and size of the premolars is not "obviously" equal to that of the molars. Another aspect that supports this theory, is an evolutionist, in which the premolars were reduced in number, the first placental mammals had four to five premolars per hemi-arch, while the primates reduced to three premolar teeth formula for hemi- arch in the Primate. In humans, were preserved two premolars per arch corresponding to the last two ontogenetically, hence they have a greater resemblance to the molars than to canines [56].

While some points of the theory of morphogenetic fields are still of extensive study and debate, in the context of dental anthropology have been conducted several studies that have allowed the characterization of morphology, so that large morphological and metric differences have been established with the molars, as the organization of the occlusal table and the number of cusps [38], concluding from the study of the frequency and variability of dental morphological traits that premolars have bilateral symmetry, there is morphological correspondence between the first and second premolars and have no sexual dimorphism [39].

3.2.4. Molars

With respect to the molar teeth, it is worth noting that these are the teeth which dental morphological features have been extensively studied in human populations, past and present. L. Aguirre et al [25] studied the correlation of morphological dental traits as cusp of Carabelli, protostylid and groove pattern between the second molars and first permanent molars of mixed Caucasoids, finding that in the first two features there is correspondence of expression and variability, bilateral symmetry and absence of sexual dimorphism, suggesting a strong genetic control. In the case of intercuspation contact pattern, there was no correspondence in the frequency and variability of the trait, which suggests that the deciduous teeth, because at higher genetic control, have retained the primitive Y or "dryopithecine " while permanent teeth, perhaps by environmental influences or by the miscegenation, tend to set a more Caucasoid + or "cruciform" pattern. This great similarity in dental morphology between the second deciduous molars and first permanent molars, reflects a common origin within the morphogenetic field, not in vain, researchers such as P. Butler and A. Dahlberg indicated that the tooth gradient deciduous and permanent molars is the second deciduous molar, since it retains the basic configuration of the contact pattern, typical of early hominids [2]. Thus, various studies have supported the theory of morphogenetic fields [61]. Later, A. Ocampo et al [62] conducted a study to determine the correlation of Carabelli, hypoconid, bridge of enamel metaconule, protostylid, elbow crease, groove pattern, number of cusps and cusp 6 and 7 between the upper and lower second molars (UM2 and LM2], the upper and lower first molars (UM1 and LM1] and second upper and lower molars (UM2 and LM2], in mixed populations of Caucasian, Afro-descendants and Colombians indigenous. Colombian indigenous are characterized by UM1/UM2/LM1/LM2 that have a high correlation with um2/lm2 in MCDT whose expression involves cusp formations (Carabelli, metaconule, groove pattern and cusp 6], suggesting high genetic conservation and low environmental influences, since these features are formed during early morphogenesis. This situation is observed in the Caucasian mestizos, but the expression of some morphological features indicates that there is more miscegenation, which may be evident in groove pattern variation from Y to +, which showed a moderate correlation. In mixed Caucasian and Afro-Colombian descent, significant correlations were observed in the same morphological features, which can be associated with their settlement in the same geographic area (southwestern Colombia) because they are part of the ethno-historical and macroevolutive processes of miscegenation [62] (Tables 1 and 2].

Teeth	Traits	Frequency (%)	Sexual dimorphysm Mann-Whitney U $p<0.05$	Bilateral simmetry Wilcoxon $p<0.05$
UI1	Winging	37.2	0.619	-
UI1/UI2	Crowding	25.4	0.481	0.428
UI1	Shovel-shape	40.1	0.697	0.157
UI2	Shovel-shape	40.9	0.269	0.829
UI1	Double shovel-shape	5.6	0.269	1.000
UM1	Carabelli trait	52.2	0.269	0.808
UM2	Carabelli trait	7.2	0.879	0.689
UM2	Hipocone reduction	65.5	0.198	0.763
LM1	Pattern cusp	3.0	0.826	0.439

Teeth	Traits	Frequency (%)	Sexual dimorphysm Mann-Whitney U p<0.05	Bilateral simmetry Wilcoxon p<0.05
LM2	Pattern cusp	7.3	0.033	0.166
LM1	Cusp number	72.4	0.630	0.491
LM2	Cusp number	40.5	0.768	0.739
LM1	Deflecting wrinkle	59.5	0.312	0.025
LM1	Protostilyd	4.2	0.072	1.000
LM2	Protostilyd	7.8	0.272	593
LM1	Cusp 6	7.8	1.000	0.271
LM2	Cusp 6	1.4	0.495	0.414
LM1	Cusp 7	15.9	0.495	0.899
LM2	Cusp 7	3.0	0.821	0.655

Table 1. Relative frequency of the non-metric dental traits al the colombian afro-descendants population

Teeth	Traits	Frequency (%)	Sexual dimorphysm Mann-Whitney U p<0.05	Bilateral simmetry Wilcoxon p<0.05
UI1	Winging	45.6	0.373	-
UI1/UI2	Crodwing	29.3	0.011	-
UI1	Shovel-shape	90.7	0.750	1.000
UI2	Shovel-shape	81.5	0.165	0.046
UI1	Double shovel-shape	20.9	0.041	0.000
UI2	Double shovel-shape	19.0	0.025	0.010
UM1	Carabelli trait	49.0	0.510	0.045
UM2	Carabelli trait	6.3	0.610	0.776
UM2	Hypocone reduction	29.4	0.405	0.527
LM1	Protostilyd	2.6	0.028	0.527
LM2	Protostilyd	4.2	0.550	0.083
LM1	Deflecting wrinkle	41.1	0.497	0.561
LM2	Deflecting wrinkle	0	0.658	0.564
LM1	Cusp pattern	17.9	0.134	0.063
LM2	Cusp pattern	12.8	0.043	0.564
LM1	Cusp number	34.8	0.704	0.180
LM2	Cusp number	36.3	0.118	0.564
LM1	Cusp 6	38.3	0.231	0.935
LM2	Cusp 6	12.5	0.299	0.063
LM1	Cusp 7	2.8	0.229	0.655
LM2	Cusp 7	0	1.000	1.000

Table 2. Relative frequency of the non-metric dental traits al the comtemporary colombian indigenous population

3.3. Statistical analysis of sexual dimorphism

Since dental morphological features are analyzed according to their expression (dichotomy presence/absence) and variability (gradation), at the time to categorize the variables for the descriptive statistical analysis, each level of expression of morphological traits constitutes a qualitative ordinal variable, where the observation methods allow to construct scales ranges from lowest to highest, according to the degree of expression [24-27].

To determine the sexual dimorphism are useful univariate nonparametric tests such as Pearson chi-square to measure the discrepancy between observed and a theoretical distribution (goodness of fit), indicating the extent to which differences between the two, if any, are due to chance in the contrast of the assumptions made in this case there is sexual dimorphism, or Mann-Whitney test, applied to two independent samples to test the two-sample heterogeneity ordinal under the null hypothesis that the distributions of departure of both distributions is the same, meaning that there is sexual dimorphism in the sample. For both tests, we adopt a $p<0.05$ in a normal distribution of the sample to reject the null hypothesis in terms of statistical significance [63].

4. Dental dimensions

Among the object of study of dental anthropology in his interest in recording, study, analyze, explain and understand the information provided by the human dentition, such as anatomical variations, developmental, pathological, cultural and therapeutic consideration with living conditions, culture, food and adaptation processes of the past and present human populations, are important the odontoscopia, the odontometry, the oral paleopathology, and modifications of the teeth. Based on this concept extensively reviewed in the literature, the odontometry or registration of dental dimensions should be studied from an interdisciplinary perspective (biology, anthropology, dentistry, paleopathology, archeology, forensics) since the teeth are the precise means to recognize individuals whose death makes it difficult to distinguish by other processes, which are part of the reconstruction of the osteobiography or odontobiography individual and general, contributing just as in estimating biological populations to clarify past its history, origin, training, contacts and movements of the past and present human groups [2,5,6,64].

Sex determination from dental measures has been one of the least developed in physical anthropology. Sex is central to this research and to help determine the taxonomic value of the traits examined [7]. The odontometry and obtaining coronal and root action of the teeth are used in different ways, depending on the interest of the study. In the dental context dimensions of the teeth are useful for the prediction of space for orthodontic treatment and orthodontics. In the anthropological context are used in comparative evolutionary studies and for establishing phylogenetic relationships among species of hominids and disappeared modern humans and to determine biological distances between populations, the same way they are used to diagnose the sex of individuals and complete paleo-demographic information of past populations. Finally, in the forensic context are useful for determining the sex of an individual in the process of identification [6,11].

Worldwide research on this topic has sheltered many of the current populations and a number of past populations, which has contributed to the elucidation of the human evolutionary processes, the population distribution in the continents of Africa, Europe and Asia, the settlement of the Americas, and the formation of population clusters by means of the dimensions of the teeth [28,29,31,40].

Since the simplification of the morphology and tooth size reduction has been the trend in the evolution of hominids, A. Zoubov -cited by J. V. Rodriguez [6]- groups the different hominid groups according to tooth size and explains them in ten points.

1. The most close to the taxonomic position Pliocene hominid are African Lothagam and Lukeino remains (6.5 and 5.5 million years), which are located in dental traits intermediate between apes and early hominids, very similar to happens to the Ardipithecus ramidus (4.4 million years ago) found in Ethiopia, whose small teeth resemble the characteristics of a chimpanzee with australopithecine cranial traits. Subsequently, the Australopithecus afarensis (3.5 million years ago) and Homo habilis (2.3 to 1.7 million years) are characterized by a higher proportion of their teeth humanoid (correlation of size between the anterior and posterior). For its part, the anterior teeth of A. africanus (3 and 2.5 million years) and A. robustus and A. boisei (2.5 to 1.5 million years) are proportionally small compared to the premolars and molars are very large. All australopithecines are characterized by molarización of the premolars and third molars large, larger than the second molars and these in turn larger than the first molars (M3> M2> M1 as meso-distal diameter).
2. Middle Pleistocene hominids such as Homo erectus, are characterized by a dental size smaller than their ancestors australopithecines but larger than in Homo sapiens. Compared to all Homo habilis had smaller teeth, excluding the lateral incisor and canine. According to the meso-distal diameter ratio had already humanoid M1> M2> M3 and harmonic proportion between the anterior and posterior teeth. Zoubov states, according to the variation of some dental traits, from that moment begin to set the division of the populations of the genus Homo into two branches: the western forms including African and European and eastern with Asian.
3. The remains known as pre-Neanderthals (450,000 and 250,000 years), labeled as archaic Homo sapiens or Neanderthal associated with late erectus or archaic, does not allow a clear division of dental dimensions and morphology, except for the presence of a bridge of enamel that connects the protoconid and metaconid of the lower molars, characteristic of European Neanderthals, indicating a relationship of genetic continuity.
4. Regarding the Neanderthals (200,000 and 35,000 years), two dental variants have been observed, a macrodonte (Krapina and Shanidar) and another microdonte (Hortus), which anyway, compared to other developmental stages, canines, premolars and molars show reduced while the incisors show an increase in size. For Asian and European Neanderthals is characteristic shovel-shape of the incisors.

5. In the case of modern humans (neoanthropus), tooth size is reduced relative to the Middle Pleistocene hominids, although with differential gradients in various regions of the world, beginning the ethnic variation over the geographic distribution of this condition. This condition increases after the Late Pleistocene, about 100,000 years ago.
6. Dental size reduction during the Late Pleistocene compared dental size between modern populations, and between the latter and the prehistoric to observe from the perspective of differences in body size, including sexual dimorphism between each taxonomic group, more evident in the canine teeth.
7. This reduction in the Upper Pleistocene dental started long before the present changes in the composition of the diet, but can be correlated with the adoption of new techniques in their preparation and use of earth ovens for cooking food, it that reduced masticatory pressure and relaxed the selection forces that remained stable during the Pleistocene. The resulting tooth reduction was the product of that C. Brace called probable mutational effect.
8. At the end of the Pleistocene the adoption of ceramics further relaxed selection forces, the beneficiaries of reduced dental system at a rate of 1% per 1,000 years. While during the Pleistocene the rate of reduction was 1% for 100,000 years, after this period was 1% for 1,000 years.
9. The maximum tooth reduction is presented in a northern strip that extends from the western to the eastern extremity. The present inhabitants of that region are the descendants of the first people to cook food.
10. To the south of the areas with oldest non-use of the teeth in the preparation of food, tooth size increases in proportion to the recent culinary skills. Homo sapiens within the lower tooth reduction are observed among the Australian Aborigines, although used as ovens on the ground for the arrival of Europeans, did not use pottery for cooking food.

First described by A. Zoubov, J. V. Rodriguez [6] argues that although tooth reduction (downsizing and streamlining of structures) was an evolutionary trend of the dental system of man, should not be understood as the loss of features, as Carabelli's tubercle and styloid formations were acquisitions undertaken in the late stages of the sapientization, as explained by the reduction theory proposed by mutational effect. Added to this, I. Shmalgausen proposes a theory about the accumulation of mutations, which holds that the simplification of the organs is a result of the uncontrolled accumulation of mutations that loosen the correlated systems during ontogenesis, in the case of the teeth, reducing the rate of growth individual body could have generated the reduction of its size, sexual dimorphism even disappearing. Other factors such as genetic isolation could produce increased tooth size, while the hybridization or miscegenation, however, could have generated reduction and simplification of the structures.

From the population point of view, the comparison of dental dimensions of different ethnic groups and those associated with the four major complexes (Australoid, Caucasoid, Mongoloid and Negroid) highlights the specificity of dental size of different populations, thus Australoids are macrodonts. Observed differences between Caucasoid and Negroid are not significant, especially labiolingual diameter of almost all teeth. The differences are more noticeable in mesiodistal diameter, particularly upper lateral incisor, premolar, second molar, mandibular canine, first premolar, first and second lower molar. The largest absolute differences are observed in the mesodistal diameter of the incisors, especially the lateral incisor, and premolars when Caucasoid and Mongoloid are compared. The Negroid reflect minor differences compared with the three major geographic and racial groups. The differences between Mongoloid and Negroid are almost nonexistent, excluding second molars [6].

4.1. Metric dental traits

The study of dental dimensions of the teeth has shown that these have a high heritability within populations worldwide. The same has been demonstrated in the study of identical twins, which is why the diameters of the crowns of the teeth have been classified as "continuous variations" whose adaptive capacity is largely related to the functions of the stomatognathic system (chewing) and detached so relative influence of the environment [56, 65,66]. Odontometric measures of the crowns of the teeth or metric dental crown traits more under study are meso-distal diameter, defined as the distance between the contact points interproximal mesial and distal and bucco-lingual diameter (lingual for lower teeth), defined as the distance between the highest convexities of the buccal and palatal (lingual) [67], because these dimensions are not affected by the wear caused by attrition during chewing or the abrasive properties of some foods [6].

For the measurements of the diameters methods used are from C. Moorrees et al [68] for meso-distal diameters (distance between the surfaces of contour mesial and distal reference plane having as the occlusal surface), in which the gauge is placed parallel or vertical to the surface occlusal so that the tips locate the areas of the mesial interproximal contact points and distal and from J. Kieser et al [69] for bucco-lingual diameters (distance between the points of greatest convex of the buccal and lingual taking as a reference plane to the occlusal surface), in which the gauge is placed parallel or vertical to the occlusal surface so that the planes of the ends locate the areas of greatest convexity of the buccal and lingual surfaces.

For individual analysis, with meso-distal dimensions and vestibule-lingual, can be calculated means as the coronal module (sum of the diameters meso-distal and bucco-lingual divided by two), the coronal index (bucco-lingual diameter multiplied by 100 and divided by the meso-distal diameter), the index of robustness of each tooth (crown area corresponds to the product of the diameters meso-distal and bucco-lingual) and the index of robustness of the dentition (sum of the indices of strength of all teeth divided by the number of types of teeth taken into account). Similarly, all these measures and indices obtained can be averaged and be applied to population analysis (frequencies, sexual dimorphism, bilateral symmetry, correspondence between metric traits within the same kind of teeth and biological distances) [12].

4.2. Sexual dimorphism and bilateral symmetry

With respect to sexual dimorphism, different authors claim that the size of the teeth is genetically determined in about 90% (64% in mesodistal diameter), so they are not affected by nutritional status or the environment. In contemporary populations has been shown that the average dimorphism with respect to meso-distal diameter is 3.1%, being canine the most dimorphic tooth. Also has been shown, from the point of view of the correspondence between the teeth of the same class that distal teeth (lateral incisor, second premolar and second molar) are the most variable [6].

The study of dental dimensions has been used to understand sexual dimorphism in the socio-ecological and phylogenetic primate evolution. Sexual dimorphism is defined as an intraspecific difference between men and women, which can be studied from the somatotype of the individual, the size and dental morphology, and correlated with patterns of intrasexual competition. During evolution, there have been ontogenetic mechanisms that cause morphological differences between males and females during primate evolution. The ontogenetic changes in these processes lead to the existence of sexual dimorphism associated with the size and evolutionary response to various factors including territoriality, competition and the distribution of resources. However, in modern humans, the restriction of many of these factors has caused the sexual dimorphism of tooth size has almost disappeared, except perhaps in the canine teeth [70].

The meso-distal and bucco-lingual teeth diameters from 100 Americans and 100 Caucasian Americans of African descent, stating that sexual dimorphism is 1.2% of the sample, while the differences between the two ethnic groups was 4.9%. The results allowed concluding that there were no significant differences between these two variables and it is difficult to establish lines of analysis given the large intra-group variations. S. Paulino et al [71] studied the dental dimensions in 153 models (115 women and 38 men) and found that there is a significant difference in the meso-distal diameter between women and men, being higher in the latter. M. Ates et al [72] determined the meso-distal and bucco-lingual diameters in a sample of 100 Turks (50 men and 50 women) and concluded that there is no sexual dimorphism in the observed sample. I. Suazo et al [73] reported that in all the permanent teeth of 150 Chilean individuals (67 men and 83 women), meso-distal and bucco-lingual diameters are higher in men, but these differences are not significant and therefore are not can consider the existence of sexual dimorphism. Astete et al [74] compared two samples of Spanish and Chilean concluding that the diameters from meso-distal and vestibulo-lingual, has a greater sexual dimorphism in Spanish than Chileans, however this difference was not statistically significant. L. Castillo et al [75] in a Colombian sample of mixed Caucasians, concluded that the meso-distal and bucco-lingual diameters are not sexually dimorphic, which was associated with the disappearance of the selective pressure of the dimorphic characteristic strength between men and women. Also these authors observed no differences in bilateral symmetry with respect to sex in the diameters of the right and left teeth in the same class, which highlights the degree of conservation of this property and its clinical significance for dental diagnosis and treatment (Table 3).

Teeth	Gender	Meso-distal diameters			Bucco-lingual diameters		
		Promedio	Standard deviation	Sexual dimorphism (p<0.05]	Promedio	Standard deviation	Sexual dimorphism (p<0.05]
UI1	Mujeres	8.368	.4619	.037	7.264	.6584	.282
	Hombres	8.653	.6211		7.068	.7690	
UI2	Mujeres	6.879	.5750	.925	6.436	.7607	.505
	Hombres	6.892	.5749		6.313	.7133	
UC	Mujeres	7.929	.7164	.897	7.754	1.0401	.804
	Hombres	7.908	.5753		7.692	.9556	
UP1	Mujeres	7.193	.7707	.779	9.679	.6641	.647
	Hombres	7.257	.7808		9.608	.5810	
UP2	Mujeres	6.900	.6128	.545	9.629	.6259	.998
	Hombres	7.003	.7198		9.629	.5229	
UM1	Mujeres	10.189	.5500	.902	11.246	.6149	.493
	Hombres	10.158	1.2567		11.335	.6479	
UI1	Mujeres	8.386	.7204	.176	7.318	.7087	.208
	Hombres	8.597	.5380		7.074	.8140	
UI2	Mujeres	6.911	.6057	.792	6.496	.7167	.314
	Hombres	6.871	.6004		6.311	.7479	
UC	Mujeres	8.036	.7004	.425	7.818	.9495	.316
	Hombres	7.916	.5144		7.603	.7786	
UP1	Mujeres	7.225	.4956	.822	9.661	.6957	.958
	Hombres	7.197	.4857		9.653	.5559	
UP2	Mujeres	6.829	.5241	.681	9.646	.7010	.721
	Hombres	6.887	.5960		9.700	.5110	
UM1	Mujeres	10.179	.5159	.112	11.164	.6510	.097
	Hombres	10.418	.6505		11.439	.6559	
LI1	Mujeres	5.225	.5001	.606	5.836	.5086	.191
	Hombres	5.284	.4265		6.000	.4926	
LI2	Mujeres	5.92	.576	.935	6.293	.6475	.520
	Hombres	5.91	.442		6.197	.5494	
LC	Mujeres	6.921	.5833	.617	7.264	.5958	.436
	Hombres	6.987	.4743		7.142	.6467	
LP1	Mujeres	7.007	.5537	.054	7.929	.6604	.385
	Hombres	7.287	.5855		8.063	.5842	
LP2	Mujeres	6.971	.6121	.078	11.404	15.2266	.326
	Hombres	7.237	.5838		8.521	.5822	
LM1	Mujeres	10.789	1.1808	.245	10.421	.6008	.593
	Hombres	11.103	.9857		10.526	.8946	
LI1	Mujeres	5.304	.3805	.850	5.936	.5599	.637

Teeth	Gender	Meso-distal diameters			Bucco-lingual diameters		
		Promedio	Standard deviation	Sexual dimorphism (p<0.05]	Promedio	Standard deviation	Sexual dimorphism (p<0.05]
	Hombres	5.324	.4553		5.997	.4949	
LI2	Mujeres	5.936	.4621	.520	6.236	.5342	.306
	Hombres	5.858	.4984		6.118	.3896	
LC	Mujeres	6.829	.6176	.571	6.943	.7781	.619
	Hombres	6.908	.5138		7.034	.6988	
LP1	Mujeres	7.218	.4423	.808	7.800	.6176	.085
	Hombres	7.245	.4409		8.056	.5613	
LP2	Mujeres	7.114	.6340	.480	8.282	.7434	.182
	Hombres	7.213	.4955		8.503	.5838	
LM1	Mujeres	11.029	.6446	.048	10.354	.6420	.033
	Hombres	11.332	.5733		10.705	.6505	

Table 3. Sexual dimorphism of the metric dental traits al the comtemporary colombian Caucasian mestizo population

4.3. Statistical analysis of sexual dimorphism

Since dental metric traits analyzed according to their measure and subsequently grouped into averages or means and standard deviations are obtained at the time to categorize the variables for the descriptive statistical analysis, each degree of expression of metric traits constitutes a quantitative ratio variable, where the observation methods for determining the measure in terms of metric units [39].

To determine the sexual dimorphism are useful parametric tests such as Student's t test to prove a hypothesis, which in this case means that if there is sexual dimorphism. It comes from a probability distribution that arises from the problem of estimating the mean of a normally distributed population when the sample size is small, considering that the observations must be independent and must be performed on normally distributed population universes whose variances groups should be homogeneous, which is not true for meso-distal diameters and vestibule-lingual, so it is necessary to previously apply the Kolmogorov-Smirnov test to determine normality and Levene to determine equality of variances . For this test, we adopt a $p < 0.05$ in a normal distribution of the sample to reject the null hypothesis in terms of statistical significance [63].

Author details

Freddy Moreno-Gómez

Dental School at the Universidad del Valle Cali, Colombia

Department of Medical Sciences at the Pontificia Universidad Javeriana Cali, Colombia

Pontificia Universidad Javeriana Cali, Colombia

5. References

[1] Rodríguez JV. Introducción a la antropología dental. Cuadernos de antropología. 1989; 19:1-41.

[2] Scott GC, Turner II CG. The anthropology of modern human teeth: dental morphology and its variation in recent human populations. First published. London: Cambridge University Press; 1997.

[3] Moreno F, Moreno SM, Díaz CA, Bustos EA, Rodríguez JV. Prevalencia y variabilidad de ocho rasgos morfológicos dentales en jóvenes de tres colegios de Cali, 2002. Colomb Med 2004; 35 (3-Supl 1):16-23.

[4] Hochrein MJ. Buried crime scene evidence: the application of forensic geotaphonomy in forensic archaeology. In forensic dentistry, Stimson PG, Mertz CA, editors. First edition. London: CRC Press; 1997.

[5] Scott GC, Turner II CG. Dental anthropology. Ann Rev Antrophol 1998; 17: 99-126.

[6] Rodríguez JV. Dientes y diversidad humana: avances de la antropología dental. Primera edición. Santa Fe de Bogotá: Universidad Nacional de Colombia; 2003.

[7] Rodríguez CD. Antropología dental prehispánica: variación y distancias biológicas en la población enterrada en el cementerio prehispánico de Obando, Valle del Cauca, Colombia entre los siglos VIII y XIII d.C. Syllaba Press. Miami. 2003.

[8] Rodríguez CD. La antropología dental y su importancia en el estudio de los grupos humanos prehispánicos. Revista de Antropología Experimental 2004; 4.

[9] Rodríguez CD. La antropología dental y su importancia en el estudio de los grupos humanos. Rev Fac Odont Univ Ant 2005; 16(1 y 2): 52-59.

[10] Marín L, Moreno F. Odontología forense: identificación odontológica, reporte de casos. Rev Estomat 2003: 11(2):41-49.

[11] Rodríguez JV. La antropología forense en la identificación humana. Universidad Nacional de Colombia. Bogotá. 2004.

[12] Hillson S. Dental anthropology. First edition. London: Cambridge University Press; 1996.

[13] Alt KW, Rosing FW, Teschler-Nicola M. Dental anthropology: fundamentals, limits, and prospects. New York: Springer-Verlag; 1998.

[14] Mayhall JT. Dental morphology: techniques and strategies. In Biological anthropology of the human skeleton, katzenberg MA, Saunders SR (Editors). Willey-Liss, New York. 2000. p. 103-134.

[15] Zoubov AA. La antropología dental y la práctica forense. Maguaré 1998; 13:243-252.

[16] Turner II CG, Nichol CR, Scott GR. Scoring procedures for key morphological traits of the permanent dentition: the Arizona State University dental anthropology system. In Nelly MA, Larsen CS (editors). Advances in dental anthropology. New York: Wiley-Liss Inc; 1991. p. 13-31.

[17] Hanihara, K. Mongoloid dental complex in the deciduous dentition. J Anthrop Soc Nippon 1966; 74: 9-20.

[18] Sciulli PW. Evolution of Dentition in Prehistoric Ohio Valley Native Americans: II. Morphology of the Deciduous Dentition. Am J Phys Anthropol 1998; 106:189-205.

[19] Grine FE. Anthropological Aspects of the Deciduous Teeth of African Blacks. En Singer L y Lundy JK (Eds) Variation, Culture and Evolution in African Populations. Johanessburg: Witwatersrand University Press. 1986. p 47-83.

[20] Nichol CR, Turner II CG. Intra and inter-observer concordance in classifying dental morphology. Am J Phys Anthropol 1986; 69:299-315.
[21] Jordan RE. Abrams L. Kraus BS. Kraus' dental anatomy and occlusion. St. Louis: Mosby; 1992
[22] Woelfel JB, Scheid RC. Dental anatomy: its relevance to dentistry, 5th ed. Baltimore: Lippincott Williams and Wilkins; 1997.
[23] Ash MM, Nelson SJ. Wheeler's dental anatomy, physiology, and occlusion. 9th ed. Philadelphia: W.B. Saunders; 2009.
[24] Moreno SM, Moreno F. Eight Non-Metric dental traits in alive racially mixed population from Cali, Colombia. Inter J Dental Anthropol 2005; 6:14-25.
[25] Aguirre L, Castillo D, Solarte D, Moreno F. Frequency and Variability of five non-metric dental crown traits in the primary and permanent dentitions of a racially mixed population from Cali, Colombia. Dental Anthropology 2006; 19(2): 39-47.
[26] Rocha L, Rivas H, Moreno F. Frecuencia y variabilidad de la morfología dental en niños afro-colombianos de una institución educativa de Puerto Tejada, Cauca, Colombia. Colomb Med 2007; 38: 210-221.
[27] Aragón N, Bastidas C, Bedón LK, Duque P, Sánchez M, Rivera S, Triana F, Noel Bedoya N, Moreno F. Rasgos morfológicos dentales coronales en dentición temporal y permanente: Distancia biológica entre tres grupos indígenas del Amazonas Colombiano. Revista Odontológica Mexicana 2008; 12(1):13-28.
[28] Hanihara T. Dental and cranial affinities among populations of East Asia and the Pacific. Am J Phys Anthropol 1992; 88:163-182.
[29] Turner II CG. Advances in the dental search for native American origins. Acta Anthropogen 1984; 8:23-78.
[30] Turner II CG. Late pleistocene and Holocene population history of East Asia based on dental variation. Am J Phys Anthropol 1987; 73:305-321.
[31] Turner II CG. Major features of sudadonty and sinodonty, including suggestions about East Asian microevolution, population history and late Pleistocene relationships with Australian aboriginals. Am J Phys Anthropol 1990; 82:295-317.
[32] Butler PM. Ontogenetic aspects of dental evolution. Int J Dev Biol 1995; 39: 25-34.
[33] Simons EL, Plavcan JM, Fleagle JG. Canine sexual dimorphism in Egyptian Eocene anthropoid primates: Catopithecus and Proteopithecus. Proc Natl Acad Sci 1999; 96:2559-62.
[34] Alba DM, Moyá-Solá S, Köhler M. Canine reduction in the Miocene hominoid Oreopithecus bambolii: behavioural and evolutionary implicationsJournal of Human Evolution 2001; 40:1-16.
[35] Plavcan JM, van Schaik CP, Kappeler PM. Competition, coalitions and canine size in primates. Journal of human evolution 1995; 28:245-276.
[36] Goyes J, Guerrero L, Narváez N, Moreno F. Rasgos morfológicos dentales coronarios de caninos temporales y permanentes en un grupo de mestizos de Cali, Colombia. Revista Colombiana de Investigación en Odontología 2011; 2(5):1-13.
[37] Irish JD, Morris DH. Technical Note: Canine Mesial Ridge (Bushman Canine) Dental Trait Definition. American Journal of Physical Anthropology 1996; 99:357-9.
[38] Nagai A, Kanazawa E. Morphological Variations of the Lower Premolars in Asian and Pacific Populations. In Dental Morphology ´98. Proceedings of the 11th International Symposium on Dental Morphology, Mayhall JT, Heikkinen T (Editors) Oulu, Finlandia; 1998. p.192-205.

[39] Girón G, Gómez P, Morales L, León M, Moreno F. Rasgos Morfológicos y Métricos Dentales Coronales de Premolares Superiores e Inferiores en Escolares de Tres instituciones Educativas de Cali, Colombia. Int J Morphol 2009; 27(3):913-925.
[40] Hanihara K. Racial characteristics in the dentition. J Anthrop Soc Japan 1967; 46: 923-926.
[41] Hanihara K. Mongoloid dental complex in the permanent dentition. Proceedings of the VIIIth International Symposium of Anthropological and Ethnological Sciences. Tokyo and Kyoto: Science Council of Japan; September 3-10, 1968. p. 298-300.
[42] Snow SR. Esthetic smile analysis of maxillary anterior tooth width: the golden percentage. Journal of Esthetic Dentistry 1999; 11(4): 177-184.
[43] Seluk LW, Brodbelt RHW, Walkera GF. Biometric comparison of face shape with denture tooth form. Journal of Oral Rehabilitation 1987; 14: 139-145
[44] Crespi R, Grossi SG. The emergence margin in prosthetic reconstruction of periodontally involved teeth. The International Journal of Periodontics & Restorative Dentistry 1993; 13(4): 349-360.
[45] Sellen P, Jagger D, Harrison A. The correlation between selected factors which influence dental aesthetics. Prim Dent Care 1998; 5(2):55-60.
[46] Ahmad I. Anterior dental aesthetics: Facial perspective. British Dental Journal 2005; 199(1):15-21.
[47] Anderson KM, Behrents RG, McKinney T, Buschang PH. Tooth shape preferences in an esthetic smile. Am J Orthod Dentofacial Orthop 2005; 128:458-65.
[48] Ibrahimagi L, V. Jerolimov V, Celebic A, Carek V, Baucic I, Knezovic-Zlataric D. Face and Tooth Form, Coll Antropol 2001; 25 (2): 619-626.
[49] Waliszewski M. Restoring dentate appearance: A literature review for modern complete denture esthetics. J Prosthet Dent 2005; 93:386-94.
[50] Berksun S, Hasanreisoğlu U, Gökdeniz B. Computer-based evaluation of gender identification and morphologic classification of tooth face and arch forms. J Prosthet Dent 2002; 88(6):578-84.
[51] Wolfart S, Menzel H, Kern M. Inability to relate tooth forms to face shape and gender. Eur J Oral Sci 2004; 112(6):471-6
[52] Acosta D, Porras A, Moreno F. Relación entre forma del contorno facial, arcos dentarios e incisivos centrales superiores en estudiantes universitarios de la ciudad de Cali Rev Estomat 2011; 19(1):14-19.
[53] Kinzey WG. Evolution of the Human Canine Tooth. American Anthropologist 1971; 73(3): 680-94.
[54] Schwartz GT, Dean C. Ontogeny of Canine Dimorphism in Extant Hominoids. Am J Phys Anthropol 2001; 115:269-83.
[55] Greenfield LO. Origin of the Human Canine: A New Solution to an Old Enigma. Yearbook of Physical Anthropology 1992; 35:153-85.
[56] van Reenen F, Reid C, Butler P. Morphological studies on human premolar crowns. In Dental Morphology ´98. Proceedings of the 11th International Symposium on Dental Morphology, Mayhall JT, Heikkinen T. (Editors) Oulu, Finlandia; 1998. p.192-205.
[57] Martinón-Torres M, Bastir M, Bermúdez de Castro JM, Gómez A, Sarmiento S, Muela A, Arsuaga JL. Hominin lower second premolar morphology: evolutionary inferences through geometric morphometric analysis. J Hum Evol 2006; 50:523-33.

[58] Harris EF. Where's the Variation? Variance Components in Tooth Sizes of the Permanent Dentition. Dental Anthropology 2003; 16(3):84-94.
[59] Moreno S, Moreno F. Antropología dental: una herramienta valiosa para fines forenses. Rev Estomat 2001; 10(2):29-42.
[60] Edgar HJH. Prediction of race using characteristics of dental morphology. J Forensic Sci 2005; 50(2):1-5.
[61] Edgar HJH, Lease LR. Correlations between deciduous and permanent tooth morphology in a european american sample. Am J Phys Anthropol 2007; 133:726-734.
[62] Ocampo AM, Sánchez JD, Martínez C, Moreno F. Correlación de diez rasgos morfológicos dentales coronales entre molares deciduos y permanentes en tres grupos étnicos colombianos. Rev Estomat 2009; 17(2):7-16.
[63] Armitage P, Berry G, Matthews JNS. Statistical methods in medical research. John Wiley & Sons: New York; 2002.
[64] Rodríguez CD, Delgado ME. Dental anthropology: a brief definition. Int J Dental Anthropol 2000; 1:2-4.
[65] Reid C, van Reenen F. Reduction in human premolar crowns. In: Dental Morphology '98. Proceedings of the 11th International Symposium on Dental Morphology, Mayhall JT, Heikkinen T. (Editors) Oulu, Finlandia; 1998. p. 85-91.
[66] Swindler DR, Drusini AG, Cristino C. & Ranzato C. Comparison of molar crown size precontact Easter Islanders with other Pacific groups. In Dental Morphology '98. Proceedings of the 11th International Symposium on Dental Morphology, Mayhall JT, Heikkinen T. (Editors) Oulu, Finlandia; 1998. p.63-73.
[67] Bernabé E, Lagravére MO, Flórez C. Permanent dentition mesio-distal and bucco-lingual crown diameters in a Peruvian sample. Inter J Dental Anthropol 2005; 6:1-13.
[68] Moorrees CFA, Thomsen SO, Jensen E, Yen PK. Mesiodistal crown diameters of the deciduous and permanent teeth in individuals. J Dent Res 1957; 36(1): 39-47.
[69] Kieser JA, Groeneveld HT, Prestosn CB. An odontometric analysis of the Lengua Indian dentition. Hum Biol 1985; 57(4): 611-620.
[70] Schwartz GT, Miller ER, Gunnell GF. Developmental processes and canine dimorphism in primate evolution. Journal of Human Evolution 2005; 48:97-103.
[71] Paulino S, Paredes-Gallardo V, Gandía-Franco JL, Cibrián-Ortiz de Anda RM. Evolución de las características de las arcadas dentarias en dos grupos de edad. RCOE 2005; 10(1):47-54.
[72] Ates M, Karaman F, Iscan M, Erdem TM. Sexual differences in Turkish dentition. Legal Medicine 2006; 8:288-292.
[73] Suazo IS, Cantín M, López F, Sandoval C, Torres S, Gajardo P, Gajardo M. Dimorfismo Sexual en las Dimensiones Mesiodistales y Bucolinguales de las Piezas Dentarias en Individuos Chilenos. Int J Morphol 2008; 26(3):609-614.
[74] Astete C, Valenzuela J, Suazo I. Sexual Dimorphism in the Tooth Dimensions of Spanish and Chilean peoples. Int J Odontostomat 2009; 3(1):47-50.
[75] Castillo L, Castro A-M, Lerma C, Lozada D, Moreno F. Diámetros meso-distales y vestíbulo-linguales dentales de un grupo de mestizos de Cali, Colombia. Rev Estomat 2012; 20(1):16-22.

Chapter 7

The Relationship Between Sexually Dimorphic Peripheral Nerves and Diseases

Hiroshi Moriyama

Additional information is available at the end of the chapter

http://dx.doi.org/10.5772/56080

1. Introduction

With regard to the incidence of peripheral nerve diseases and peripheral nerve damage after surgical procedures, there are reports of sexual dimorphism, no sexual dimorphism, and little sexual dimorphism. However, details of the morphology and sexual dimorphism in the characteristics of peripheral nerves have not been available in textbooks. I morphometrically analyzed peripheral nerves and clarified these issues.

2. Materials and methods

The materials used in this study were Japanese oculomotor nerves, ophthalmic nerves, inferior alveolar nerves, abducent nerves, facial nerves, vestibular nerves, cochlear nerves, and vagus nerves, recurrent laryngeal nerves in the cranial nerve group; Japanese femoral nerves and tibial nerves in the spinal nerve group; and Japanese greater splanchnic nerves and lesser splanchnic nerves in the autonomic nerve group. All the cadavers were donated with the individual's consent. We proceeded to perform this research in accordance with the law concerning autopsy and preservation of corpses, and concerning donation for medical and dental education. In no case was there a history of peripheral nerve disorders such as neuroparalysis or schwannoma, or of treatment with toxic agents or irradiation therapy. The causes of death did not directly or indirectly influence the nervous system, so the peripheral nerves were considered to be normal. I used right side specimens of right-handed persons to avoid any interaction between the effects of sex and side. Moreover, the age of specimens showed no significant difference between female and male specimens. The data on the above pairs of groups were thus independent of the aging process. The methods for preparation of sections, also described in our previous report [1], were as follows:

2.1. Fixation

The fixation involved a two-step process. For the first step, all the cadavers were fixed with a 10% solution of formalin (3.7% formaldehyde) within 24 h postmortem. After resecting the peripheral nerves, a 10% solution of formalin (3.7% formaldehyde) was used for immersion for at least a week. The solution was changed once in the first 30–60 min and again, later if desired.

The formalin-fixed materials were then transferred without washing to the secondary fixative (1:4 mixture of 5% $K_2Cr_2O_7$ and 5% K_2CrO_4) and maintained at room temperature for 2 weeks. If the solution became turbid or precipitated it was changed. After this, the fixation was continued at 37°C for an additional week. The volume of fixative used was at least ten times the volume of the specimens.

2.2. Washing

The fixed materials were washed in running water for around 24 h. We used a siphon-operated automatic pipette washer with the materials packed in a small plastic basket.

2.3. Dehydration and celloidin embedding

1. 50% ethanol, for several days
2. 70% ethanol, for several days

The alcohol in steps 1 and 2 was changed if it became yellow.

3. 90% ethanol, overnight
4. 95% ethanol, overnight
5. Pure ethanol, one night or more
6. Ether/ethanol, 1:1 overnight
7. 1% celloidin in ether/ethanol, several days
8. 7% celloidin, several days
9. 14% celloidin for embedding, several weeks
10. Immerse hardened celloidin embedded blocks in 90–95% ethanol for several hours
11. Maintained celloidin blocks in 70% ethanol prior to sectioning

2.4. Staining procedures

Modified luxol fast blue-periodic acid Schiff-hematoxylin (LPH) triple stain.

1. Cut sections 15 μm thick and place in 90% ethanol
2. Rinse sections in 95% ethanol
3. Keep at 58°C overnight in LFB solution (0.1% solution of luxol fast blue by dissolving 1.0 g of the substance in 1,000 ml of 95% ethanol) placed in a shallow sealed jar.
4. Immerse in 95% ethanol and wash off excess stain
5. Wash in distilled water

6. Differentiate in 2% saturated lithium carbonate (= 0.03% Li_2CO_3) for 60 min
7. Continue differentiation with one or two changes of 70% ethanol until myelin sheaths can be distinguished. If necessary, repeat steps 5 through 7 until there is sharp contrast between myelin sheaths and surrounding structures.
8. Finish differentiation by rinsing in 95% ethanol
9. Wash in distilled water (two changes)
10. Oxidize for 5 min in 0.5% periodic acid
11. Wash in distilled water (several changes)
12. Immerse for 15 min in Schiff's reagent
13. Immediately transfer to 5% sodium hydrogen sulfite and leave for about 5 min, changing the solution three times
14. Wash in distilled water (several changes)
15. Immerse sections for around 5 min in Mayer's hematoxylin solution
16. Wash sections in distilled water (several changes) until sections turn bluish.
17. Rinse in 90–95% ethanol
18. Dehydrate sections in *n*-butyl alcohol (three changes)
19. Clear sections in xylene (three changes)
20. Mount in balsam

2.5. Morphometry

I observed the fascicles at low power (Fig. 1). I covered the entire area of the distributed myelinated axons in the peripheral nerve by moving the eyepiece grid vertically and horizontally. I confirmed that I could distinguish myelinated structures from vessels in the tissue with a computer or grouped unmyelinated axons with the naked eye in each grid. I counted the myelinated axons and measured the transverse area and perimeter of the myelinated axons in a square eyepiece grid at high power (Fig. 2). To avoid duplicate counts, I counted and measured all axons on the side of the grid that did not come into contact with the other grids. In the case of grids adjacent to the other grids, I counted and measured only the axons on the lower right side of the grid, not those on the upper left side. I used a microscope in transmitted light mode (BX50, Olympus, Tokyo, Japan) equipped with a high-resolution digital camera (ColorView12, Soft Imaging System, Münster, Germany), a motorized XYZ stage (Märzhäuser, Wetzlar-Steindorf, Germany), a stage controller (Märzhäuser, Wetzlar-Steindorf, Germany), and a computer (Precision 530, Dell, Austin, TX, USA) with analyzing system software (analySIS 3.0, Soft Imaging System, Münster, Germany) to store data on-line, do calculations, and perform statistical analyses. Circularity ratios (CR) were calculated as follows: $CR = 4\pi A/L^2$ (A = area in mm^2; L = perimeter in mm).

If a circle is regular, the ratio has a maximum value of 1.0, and if it is irregular, the value is less than 1. This indicates how near or far each irregularity is from a regular round figure, allowing quantitative comparison of round figures.

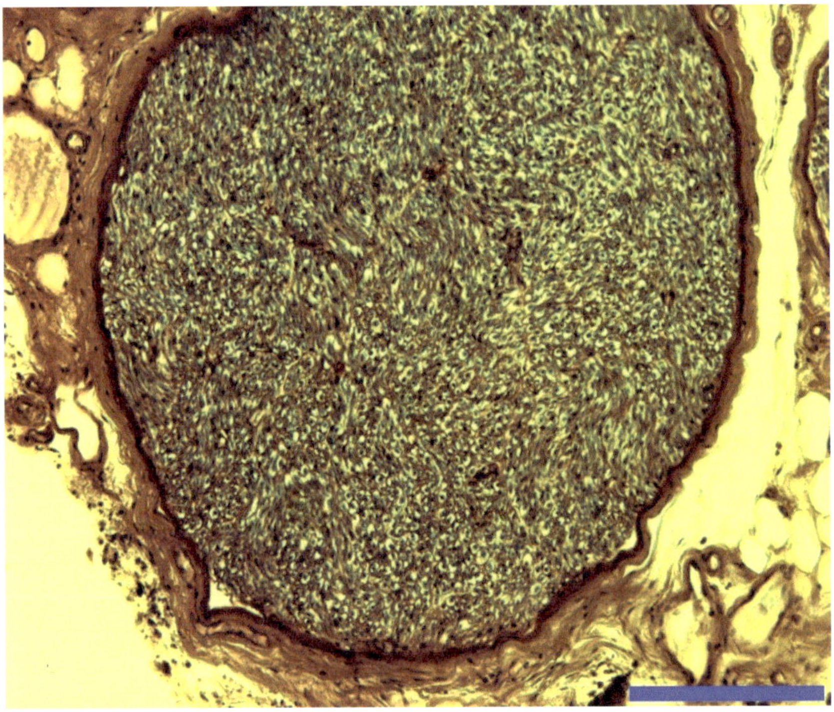

Figure 1. A low-power view of the inferior alveolar nerve from a 65-year-old woman, modified LPH stain. *Scale bar* 200 μm

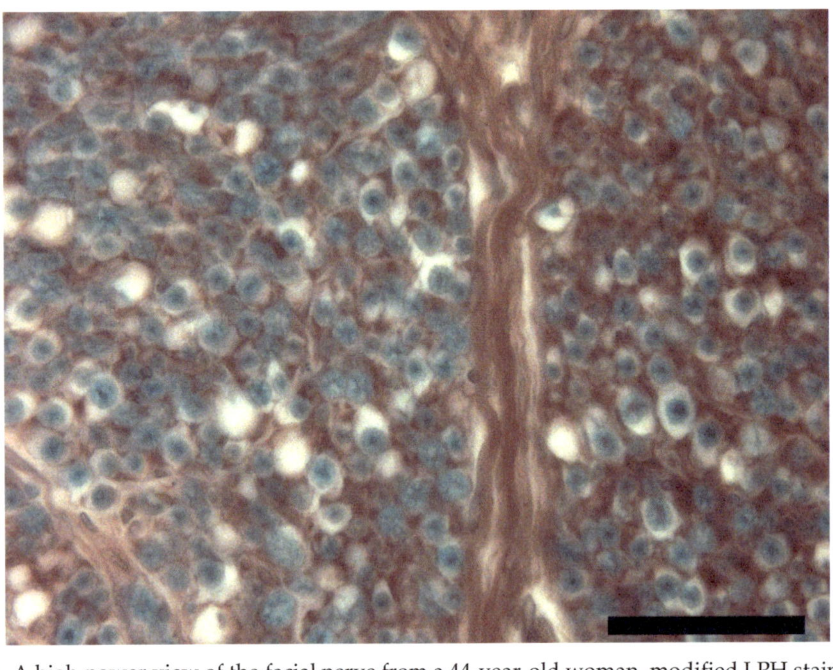

Figure 2. A high-power view of the facial nerve from a 44-year-old woman, modified LPH stain. Axons were stained *dark purple or black*, and surrounded by a myelin sheath stained *deep green*. Scale bar 50 μm

2.6. Statistical analyses

All statistical analyses were performed using JMP statistical software version 9.0.3 (SAS Institute Inc. Cary, NC, USA) on a Macintosh personal computer.

Researchers have studied shrinkage of embedding materials, and found that celloidin and plastination embedding exhibit less shrinkage (around 10%) than paraffin and other embeddings [2]. Therefore, although I measured every myelinated axon, I calculated the average transverse area and perimeter of myelinated axons after excluding data far from the median (15%) due to shrinkage.

Morphological differences between female and male specimens were analyzed by applying a parametric unpaired t test (where data were normally distributed with equal variance) to the total number of myelinated axons and the average transverse area, perimeter and CR. A p value of <0.05 was considered to indicate a statistically significant difference.

3. Results

3.1. Number of myelinated axons

We estimated the total number or number per unit area of myelinated axons (NM) in the peripheral nerves (Table 1). The myelinated nerve fibers appeared as a blue-green myelin sheath surrounding a dark purple or black axon (Fig. 2). According to the data, there was no statistically significant difference in the total number of myelinated axons between the female and male specimens of the peripheral nerves, except for the vestibular nerve ($P < 0.05$; Table 1).

3.2. Average transverse area of myelinated axons

The average transverse area of myelinated axons (ATA) in the peripheral nerves was calculated (Table 1). According to the data, there was no statistically significant difference in the average transverse area of myelinated axons between the female and male specimens of all calculated peripheral nerves ($P < 0.05$; Table 1).

3.3. CR of myelinated axons

The average CR of myelinated axons (ACR) in the peripheral nerves was calculated (Table 1) and there was no statistically significant difference in the average CR of myelinated axons between the female and male specimens of the peripheral nerves, except for the vagus nerve ($P < 0.05$; Table 1).

4. Discussion

Researchers have reported that a decrease in the number and size of myelinated axons influences the occurrence of peripheral nerve palsy or neuropathy [3-6], and a lower CR of myelinated axons has been partly implicated in the degeneration of nerve fibers [7]. A smaller NM, ATA, and lower ACR of myelinated axons would help explain the sex difference in the incidence of peripheral nerve palsy and neuropathy.

Nerve	Side	Sex	Number of Specimens	Age	Total Number or Number /Unit area	Average Transverse Area (μm²)	Average Circularity Ratio
Oculomotor	R	F	10	70.8 ± 8.6	18,905 ± 4,861	5.59 ± 1.54	0.83 ± 0.07
	R	M	10	72.5 ± 8.9	18,523 ± 5,700	6.28 ± 1.95	0.83 ± 0.06
		p value		P=0.65	P=0.79	P=0.62	P=0.82
		95% CI		−6.5 to 9.9	−5,359 to 4,595	−0.97 to 2. 34	−0.06 to 0.06
Ophthalmic	R	F	22	75.2 ± 13.8	34 ± 11 / 16×16 μm²	4.86 ± 2.27	0.83 ± 0.05
	R	M	22	73.3 ± 15.7	36 ± 7 / 16×16 μm²	4.88 ± 1.38	0.84 ± 0.06
		p value		P=0.82	P=0.47	P=0.94	P=0.65
		95% CI		−15.8 to 12.0	−7 to 11	−1.75 to 1.79	−0.04 to 0.07
Inferior Alveolar	R	F	11	72.5 ± 8.6	21,885 ± 7,711	34.90 ± 8.97	0.87 ± 0.03
	R	M	11	75.6 ± 7.3	23,623 ± 6,684	30.95 ± 8.76	0.86 ± 0.05
		p value		P=0.32	P=0.55	P=0.62	P=0.77
		95% CI		−4.0 to 10. 2	−4,680 to 8,157	−11.84 to 3.93	−0.05 to 0.03
Abducent	R	F	10	73.8 ± 7.4	1,854 ± 343	4.34 ± 0.75	0.80 ± 0.08
	R	M	10	75.6 ± 9.3	2,139 ± 502	3.46 ± 0.50	0.76 ± 0.06
		p value		P=0.68	P=0.40	P=0.09	P=0.75
		95% CI		−10.5 to 14. 1	−341 to 911	−1.81 to 0.05	−0.14 to 0.07
Facial	R	F	10	65.9 ± 15.9	6,023 ± 955	6.34 ± 0.92	0.80 ± 0.04
	R	M	10	65.1 ± 15.2	6,466 ± 735	6.27 ± 0.74	0.79 ± 0.03
		p value		P=0.91	P=0.26	P=0.86	P=0.85
		95% CI		−13.8 to 15.4	−357 to 1,244	−0.71 to 0.85	−0.13 to 0.10
Vestibular	R	F	12	75.4 ± 9.6	18,022 ± 2,780 *	3.76 ± 0.65	0.88 ± 0.03
	R	M	12	74.2 ± 10.2	21,002 ± 4,636 *	3.56 ± 0.93	0.86 ± 0.08
		p value		P=0.69	P=0.04	P=0.56	P=0.93
		95% CI		−9.7 to 7. 2	−256 to 6,217	−0.88 to 0.48	−0.07 to 0.03
Cochlear	R	F	12	68.7 ± 18.0	23,597 ± 5,377	1.81 ± 0.40	0.86 ± 0.01
	R	M	12	72.0 ± 17.9	26,598 ± 6,177	1.78 ± 0.30	0.86 ± 0.02
		p value		P=0.75	P=0.30	P=0.69	P=0.62
		95% CI		−19.7 to 26.4	−4,449 to 10,450	−0.48 to 0.43	−0.02 to 0.01
Vagus	R	F	15	75.9 ± 15.4	1,413 ± 274	1.12 ± 0.33	0.79 ± 0.06 *
	R	M	15	77.8 ± 11.2	1,331 ± 192	1.21 ± 0.30	0.83 ± 0.06 *
		p value		P=0.79	P=0.72	P=0.57	P=0.03
		95% CI		−8.1 to 11.9	−257 to 94	−0.15 to 0.32	−0.00 to 0.09
Recurrent Laryngeal	R	F	10	78.7 ± 10.2	14 ± 2 / 33×33 μm²	10.06 ± 3.15	0.88 ± 0.04
	R	M	10	73.0 ± 8.8	14 ± 3 / 33×33 μm²	10.38 ± 2.57	0.89 ± 0.06
		p value		P=0.28	P=0.96	P=0.96	P=0.51
		95% CI		−15.5 to 5. 3	−3 to 3	−2.77 to 3.41	−0.05 to 0.08
Femoral	R	F	10	83.7 ± 9.9	26.7 ± 11.7	5.06 ± 1.54	0.93 ± 0.08
	R	M	10	76.4 ± 11.8	30.4 ± 10.9	6.09 ± 1.84	0.92 ± 0.07
		p value		P=0.31	P=0.52	P=0.31	P=0.70
		95% CI		−20.0 to 5.4	−9.5 to 16.9	−0.94 to 3.01	−0.09 to 0.07
Tibial	R	F	10	84.9 ± 12.3	1,023 ± 680	2.60 ± 0.39	0.94 ± 0.05
	R	M	10	82.5 ± 9.9	1,491 ± 1,061	3.20 ± 0.75	0.90 ± 0.09
		p value		P=0.61	P=0.72	P=0.07	P=0.57
		95% CI		−16.2 to 11.5	−602 to 1,538	−0.11 to 1.31	−0.12 to 0.05

Nerve	Side	Sex	Number of Specimens	Age	Total Number or Number /Unit area	Average Transverse Area (μm²)	Average Circularity Ratio
Greater Splanchnic	R	F	15	73.3 ± 15.6	8 ± 2 / 16×16 μm²	5.18 ± 1.36	0.88 ± 0.07
	R	M	15	72.9 ± 12.1	9 ± 2 / 16×16 μm²	5.54 ± 1.26	0.87 ± 0.06
		p value		P=0.93	P=0.43	P=0.35	P=0.71
		95% CI		−10.8 to 10.0	−1 to 2	−0.62 to 1.33	−0.06 to 0.04
Lesser Splanchnic	R	F	15	73.7 ± 15.5	12 ± 6 / 16×16 μm²	1.63 ± 0.96	0.85 ± 0.10
	R	M	15	72.1 ± 12.5	14 ± 7 / 16×16 μm²	1.55 ± 0.62	0.86 ± 0.11
		p value		P=0.66	P=0.43	P=0.88	P=0.96
		95% CI		−12.3 to 9.1	−3 to 8	−0.67 to 0.52	−0.08 to 0.10

* Indicates a significant difference ($p < 0.05$).
Each value is the mean ± SD
CI confidence interval

Table 1. Nerve fiber analysis of peripheral nerves in humans.

4.1. Oculomotor nerve

Cabrejas et al. reported epidemiological data on oculomotor nerve palsy that there were 59.1% males, with no statistically significant difference between females and males ($p = 0.574$) [8]. Moreover, Ohguro et al. reported finding differences in oculomotor nerve palsy with causative disease incidence according to sex, but they reported finding no significant difference in oculomotor nerve palsy with unknown cause incidence according to sex [9]. According to the data in this study, there was no statistically significant difference in the NM, ATA, or ACR of myelinated axons between the female and male specimens of the oculomotor nerve ($P < 0.05$; Table 1). My findings may partly explain why there is no significant sex difference in the incidence of oculomotor nerve palsy.

4.2. Ophthalmic nerve

Researchers have reported that the incidence rate of trigeminal neuralgia (TN) was slightly higher for females than for males. For example, the female-to-male ratio was 1.74:1 in the Katusic et al. study [10] and 3:2 in another study by Ashkenazi and Levin [11]. It has been proposed that the symptoms of TN are caused by demyelination of the nerve leading to ephaptic transmission of impulses. Surgical specimens have demonstrated this demyelination and close apposition of demyelinated axons in the trigeminal root of patients with TN [12]. Results from experimental studies suggest that demyelinated axons are prone to ectopic impulses, which may transfer from light touch to pain fibers in close proximity (ephaptic conduction) [12]. Current theories regarding the cause of this demyelination center on vascular compression of the nerve root by aberrant or tortuous vessels. Accepting current theories, neurovascular (or microvascular) decompression, when a pad is placed between a vessel and the nerve, has been found empirically to be an effective treatment for TN in cases resistant to medical therapy, and as many as 90% of cases have been relieved [13-15]. Barker et al. reported that 706 patients (around 60%) were female of 1185 patients who underwent microvascular decompression, and female sex was a risk factor for recurrence after microvascular decompression (hazard ratio 1.3; $P = 0.06$) [16]. According to the data here, there was no statistically significant difference in the NM, ATA, or ACR of myelinated axons between the female and male specimens of the ophthalmic nerve ($P < 0.05$; Table 1). Therefore, a vascular abnormality in the female TN may be one reason why TN has a female preponderance, but morphology in the characteristic nerve does not appear to explain the sex difference in the incidence of TN.

4.3. Inferior alveolar nerve

Inferior alveolar nerve (IAN) damage can occur after an IAN block [17, 18] or following oral and maxillofacial surgical procedures [19-24]. With regard to the incidence of IAN damage after these procedures, Haas and Lennon reported no significant sex difference (ratio of affected females to males, 72:68) [25]. Kipp et al. also reported that the incidence was 7% in both sexes, indicating no significant sex difference [26], while Harn and Durham reported that there was little sex difference in postinjection lingual nerve injuries (ratio of affected females to males, 24:17) [27]. Meanwhile, sexual dimorphism that results in the incidence being almost twice as high in females than in males has been reported [17, 28, 29]. Pogrel and Thamby [17] found the difference in referral rates for male and female patients difficult to explain. They mentioned that there have been studies suggesting that nerves respond differently to injury in female animals than in male animals [30]. Coyle et al. [31] reported that female rats were more prone to developing tactile allodynia than male rats after partial sciatic nerve ligation. These reports [30, 31] may partially explain the indicated sex difference in the incidence of IAN damage. According to this study's data, there was no statistically significant difference in the NM, ATA, or ACR of myelinated axons between the female and male IAN specimens ($P < 0.05$; Table 1). Heasman and Beynon [32] reported a difference between the total number of myelinated axons in the human IAN of dentate and edentulous groups as significant ($P < 0.001$) and suggested axonal atrophy in the main nerve trunk following tooth loss. As each cadaver in this study had 7 teeth (central incisor, lateral incisor, canine, first premolar, second premolar, first molar, and second molar) on the side of the mandible that I used, I considered that this result was not affected by the dentulous condition. Therefore, the results of this study suggest a nonsignificant sex difference in the incidence of IAN damage, supported by the morphometric analysis. These findings may partly explain why there is no significant sex difference in the incidence of IAN damage.

4.4. Abducent nerve

Patel et al. reported 69 male (50%) and 68 female (50%) cases of abducent nerve palsy or paresis [33]. According to this study, ATA in the female abducent nerve was larger than that in the male abducent nerve, but there was no statistically significant difference in the NM, ATA, or ACR of myelinated axons between the female and male specimens of the oculomotor nerve ($P < 0.05$; Table 1). My findings may partly explain why there is no significant sex difference in the incidence of abducent nerve palsy or paresis.

4.5. Facial nerve

Campbell and Brundage [34] reported that the incidence rate of Bell's palsy (BP) was slightly higher for females than for males (rate ratio = 1.16). Meanwhile, Monini et al. [35] reported that males were slightly more affected (53.7%) than females. However, many researchers have reported finding no significant difference in BP incidence according to sex, as Tiemstra and Khatkhate [36] recently reported. In this study, there was no statistically significant difference in the NM, ATA, or ACR of myelinated axons between the female and male facial nerve specimens ($P < 0.05$; Table 1). These findings may partly explain why there is no significant sex difference in the incidence of BP.

4.6. Vestibular nerve

The incidence of vestibular dysfunction has a female preponderance in a textbook description [37]. There was a marked female preponderance among individuals with vestibular vertigo (one year prevalence ratio female to male of 2.7:1.0) [38]. Neuhauser et al. also reported that prevalence and incidence rates of vestibular vertigo were consistently higher in females than in males, for example, the lifetime prevalence ratio of female to male was 10.3:4.3, and the population incidence ratio (one year) female to male was 1.9:0.8 [39]. This female preponderance tended to increase with age [40]. Yin et al. reported that adults (18-65y) had a ratio of affected females to males of 59.1:40.9, but elderly adults (>65y) had a ratio of 60.6:39.4 [40]. With regard to Menière's disease, a female preponderance can be assumed based on the data from Rochester (61% women) [41] and is confirmed by the latest data from Finland [42]. The results here showed that NM was 2,980 (mean value) higher in the male vestibular nerve than the female vestibular nerve. My data also indicated a significant sex difference ($P = 0.04$; Table 1), but there was no statistically significant difference in the ATA and ACR of myelinated axons between the female and male vestibular nerve specimens ($P < 0.05$; Table 1). The lower NM of myelinated axons in the female vestibular nerve may be one of the reasons why vestibular disorders have a female preponderance, but the findings here on ATA and ACR of myelinated axons did not appear to explain the sex difference in the incidence of these diseases.

4.7. Cochlear nerve

There are some reports regarding the incidence of cochlear dysfunction with sex difference. The incidence of tinnitus has a female preponderance in a textbook description [43]. Meanwhile, Graham [44] and the National Study of Hearing [45] reported that the incidence rate of tinnitus was higher for females than for males until the mid-fifties, but after the mid-fifties, that of tinnitus was higher for males than for females. Møller et al. reported that of the 72 patients who underwent microvascular decompression of the intracranial portion of the auditory nerve, 54.8% experienced total relief from tinnitus or marked improvement [46]. This report indicated that vascular compression of the auditory nerve was a factor in tinnitus. Therefore, vascular abnormalities in tinnitus patients may be one reason why tinnitus shows a sex difference, but morphology in the characteristic nerve does not appear to explain the sex difference in the incidence of tinnitus. Next, with regard to the incidence of hearing acuity, Kacker reported that there was no significant sex difference [47]. Meanwhile, Hinchcliffe and Jones reported that the hearing acuity in males was better than that in females [48]. Researchers also reported that the differences in hearing levels between females and males depended on the frequencies or race [49, 50]. Moreover, Star et al. reported that there were four females and six males among 10 patients with auditory nerve disease [51]. The main lesion in auditory nerve disease is thought to be demyelination or degeneration of cochlear nerve fibers. Finally, Nakashima examined the nationwide epidemiological study of sudden deafness in 1993, and reported that there was no significant sex difference [52]. In this study, there was no statistically significant difference in the NM, ATA, or ACR of myelinated axons between the female and male cochlear nerve specimens ($P < 0.05$; Table 1). The findings here may partly explain why there is no significant sex difference in the incidence of cochlear dysfunction.

4.8. Vagus nerve

Araújo et al. assessed vagal activity using heart rate response to a short (4s) bicycle exercise test during maximal inspiratory apnea. This study aimed to evaluate the role of sex and physical activity patterns on vagal activity. As a result, no sex effect could be identified [53]. With regard to vagoglossopharyngeal neuralgia, researchers reported that there was no preponderance regarding sex [54, 55]. I gave a supplementary explanation for the term "vagoglossopharyngeal neuralgia". As researchers took the central or peripheral overlap between the glossopharyngeal nerve and vagus nerve into consideration, they grouped glossopharyngeal and vagal neuralgia together, and used the more useful vagoglossopharyngeal neuralgia in clinical practice [56, 57]. Meanwhile, Khasar et al. reported that under normal conditions, responses to noxious stimuli were modulated by vagus nerve activity in males, but not in females [58]. My results showed that ACR was 0.04 (mean value) higher in the male vagus nerve than the female vagus nerve. My data also indicated a significant sex difference ($P = 0.03$; Table 1). However, there was no statistically significant difference in the NM and ATA of myelinated axons between the female and male vagus nerve specimens ($P < 0.05$; Table 1). The higher ACR of myelinated axons in the male vagus nerve may be one reason why vagus nerve activity to modulate pain has a male preponderance. My findings regarding the NM and ATA of myelinated axons may partly explain why there is no significant sex difference in the incidence of vagoglossopharyngeal neuralgia.

4.9. Recurrent laryngeal nerve

With respect to sex, males with recurrent laryngeal nerve paralysis were more frequent than females in some reports [59-65] whereas in some other reports [66-68], there were more females than males with that condition. However, overall the above data indicated that there were 1,526 females with recurrent laryngeal nerve paralysis (48.5%) and 1,618 males (51.5%) [64]. Therefore, there was no significant difference in the number of patients between the two sexes. In this study, there was no statistically significant difference in the NM, ATA, or ACR of myelinated axons between the female and male recurrent laryngeal nerve specimens ($P < 0.05$; Table 1). These findings may partly explain why there is no significant sex difference in the incidence of recurrent laryngeal nerve paralysis.

4.10. Femoral and tibial nerve

Shinoda analyzed data on adult motor neuropathy in past reports, and mentioned that the vulnerability of male motor neurons was higher than that of female motor neurons [69]. With regard to amyotrophic lateral sclerosis (ALS), a progressive disorder of motor neurons, the incidence of ALS was slightly higher for males than for females (male/female rate was 2.0% or less) in reports including 100 cases or more. For example, Collins [70], Bonduelle et al. [71], Boman and Meurman [72], Erbslöh et al. [73], Kondo [74], and Haberlandt [75] reported that the male/female rate ratio was 1.1, 1.2, 1.3, 1.5, 1.5, 2.0, respectively. According to my data, there was no statistically significant difference in the NM, ATA, or ACR of myelinated axons between the female and male femoral and tibial nerve specimens ($P < 0.05$; Table 1). These findings may partly explain why there is little significant sex difference in the incidence of motor neuropathy. Therefore, sex difference in the incidence of motor neuropathy is considered to be caused not only due to the morphology of the motor neurons, but also because of sex hormones and other factors.

4.11. Greater splanchnic and lesser splanchnic nerve

Shinoda analyzed data on adult autonomic neuropathy in past reports and mentioned that the vulnerability of male autonomic neurons was higher than that of females [69]. Hogarth and coworkers' study demonstrated that females have a lower central sympathetic nerve activity to the periphery, the mechanism of which involves a greater baroreceptor reflex inhibitory effect on this activity in females than in males [76]. These findings could have implications regarding the lower number of cardiovascular events observed in females than in males. Muneta et al. reported that the activation of the sex center regulating gonadotropin secretion may be a causative factor in the baroreflex impairment in females [77]. They also mentioned that changes in blood pressure in females are more sensitive to mental stress, but less so to isometric stress than those of males. These findings suggest that ovarian dysfunction is another important factor influencing the baroreflex function in addition to aging and blood pressure, and that the baroreflex impairment in females characterizes the sex difference in the pathophysiology of essential hypertension. Hinojosa-Laborde et al. reported that clear evidence exists for differences in the regulation of the sympatho-adrenal nervous system between males and females [78]. At each level of neural control examined in their review, females were able to limit the activation or enhance the inhibition of the sympathetic nervous system (SNS) more effectively than males during at least part of the oestral/menstrual cycle. These observations suggest that the ability of females to more tightly control the SNS and, subsequently, arterial pressure may serve as a mechanism whereby sex hormones protect females against hypertension. Here, there was no statistically significant difference in the NM, ATA, or ACR of myelinated axons between the female and male specimens of the greater splanchnic and lesser splanchnic nerve ($P < 0.05$; Table 1). These findings do not explain why there is a significant sex difference in the incidence of autonomic dysfunction. Therefore, the morphology of autonomic neurons may not be the cause of sex differences in the incidence of autonomic dysfunction and other factors such as sex hormones may be the cause.

Author details

Hiroshi Moriyama
Showa University School of Medicine, Japan

Acknowledgement

We thank Ms. Ikuko Moriyama for assistance in preparing the manuscript. This work was supported by a Grant-in-aid for Scientific Research B14370007 from the Ministry of Education, Culture, Sports, Science and Technology of Japan.

5. References

[1] Moriyama H, Amano K, Itoh M, Shimada K, Otsuka N (2007) Morphometric aspects of peripheral nerves in adults and the elderly. J Peripher Nerv Syst 12:205–209

[2] Eckel HE, Sittel C, Walger M, Sprinzl G, Koebke J (1993) Plastination: a new approach to morphological research and instruction with excised larynges. Ann Otol Rhinol Laryngol 102:660–665

[3] Fukuda M, Morimoto T, Suzuki Y, Kida K, Ohnishi A (2000) Congenital neuropathy with the absence of large myelinated fibers. Pediatr Neurol 23:349–351

[4] Griffn JW, Höke A (2005) The control of axonal caliber. In: Dyck PJ, Thomas PK (eds) Peripheral Neuropathy, 4th edn, vol 1. Elsevier Saunders, Philadelphia, pp 433–446

[5] Korinthenberg R, Sauer M, Ketelsen UP, Hanemann CO, Stoll G, Graf M, Baborie A, Volk B, Wirth B, Rudnik-Schoneborn S, Zerres K (1997) Congenital axonal neuropathy caused by deletions in the spinal muscular atrophy region. Ann Neurol 42:364–368

[6] Lin KP, Soong BW (2002) Peripheral neuropathy of Machado-Joseph disease in Taiwan: a morphometric and genetic study. Eur Neurol 48:210–217

[7] Moriyama H, Shimada K, Goto N (1995) Morphometric analysis of neurons in ganglia: geniculate, submandibular, cervical spinal and superior cervical. Okajimas Folia Anat Jpn 72:185–190

[8] Cabrejas L, Hurtado-Ceña FJ, Tejedor J (2009) Predictive factors of surgical outcome in oculomotor nerve palsy. J AAPOS 13:481-484

[9] Ohguro H, Takeda M, Nakagawa T (1986) Acquired oculomotor nerve palsy: A review of 74 cases. Neuro-ophthalmol Jpn 3:263-266 (Japanese)

[10] Katusic S, Beard CM, Bergstralh E, Kurland LT (1990) lncidence and clinical features of trigeminal neuralgia, Rochester, Minnesota, 1945–1984. Ann Neurol 27:89–95

[11] Ashkenazi A, Levin M (2004) Three common neuralgias. How to manage trigeminal, occipital, and postherpetic pain. Postgrad Med 116:16–32

[12] Love S, Coakham HB (2001) Trigeminal neuralgia: pathology and pathogenesis [published correction appears in Brain. 2002;125:687]. Brain 124:2347-2360

[13] Apfelbaum R (1988) Surgical management of disorders of the lower cranial nerves. In: Schmideck H, Sweet W, (eds) Operative neurosurgical techniques. 2nd edn, Grune & Stratton, New York, pp. 1097-1109

[14] Wilkins RH (1988) Surgical therapy of neuralgia: Vascular decompression procedures. Semin Neurol 8:280–285

[15] Jannetta PJ (1990) Cranial rhizopathies. In: Youmans JR (ed) Neurological surgery. 3rd edn, WB Saunders, Philadelphia, pp. 4169–4182

[16] Barker FG II, Jannetta PJ, Bissonette DJ, Larkins MV, Jho HD (1996) The long-term outcome of microvascular decompression for trigeminal neuralgia. N Engl J Med 334:1077-83

[17] Pogrel MA, Thamby S (2000) Permanent nerve involvement resulting from inferior alveolar nerve blocks. J Am Dent Assoc 131:901-907

[18] Lambrianidis T, Molyvdas J (1987) Paresthesia of the inferior alveolar nerve caused by periodontal-endodontic pathosis. Oral Surg Oral Med Oral Pathol 63:90-92

[19] Pogrel MA, Bryan J, Regezi J (1995) Nerve damage associated with inferior alveolar nerve blocks. J Am Dent Assoc 126:1150-1155

[20] Giuliani M, Lajolo C, Deli G, Silveri C (2001) Inferior alveolar nerve paresthesia caused by endodontic pathosis: A case report and review of the literature. Oral Surg Oral Med Oral Pathol Oral Radiol Endod 92:670-674

[21] Panula K, Finne K, Oikarinen K (2001) Incidence of complications and problems related to orthognathic surgery: A review of 655 patients. J Oral Maxillofac Surg 59:1128-1136

[22] Blanas N, Kienle F, Sàndor GKB (2002) Injury to the Inferior alveolar nerve due to thermoplastic gutta percha. J Oral Maxillofac Surg 60:574-576

[23] Kraut RA, Chahal O (2002) Management of patients with trigeminal nerve injuries after mandibular implant placement. J Am Dent Assoc 133:1351-1354

[24] Teerijoki-Oksa T, Jääskeläinen S, Forssell K, Virtanen A, Forssell H (2003) An evaluation of clinical and electrophysiology tests in nerve injury diagnosis after mandibular sagittal split osteotomy. Int J Oral Maxillofac Surg 32:15-23

[25] Haas DA, Lennon D (1995) A 21 year retrospective study of reports of paresthesia following local anesthetic administration. J Can Dent Assoc 61:319- 320, 323-326, 329-330

[26] Kipp DP, Goldstein BH, Weiss WW Jr (1980) Dysesthesia after mandibular third molar surgery: A retrospective study and analysis of 1,377 surgical procedures. J Am Dent Assoc 100:185-192

[27] Harn SD, Durham TM (1990) Incidence of lingual nerve trauma and postinjection complications in conventional mandibular block anesthesia. J Am Dent Assoc 121:519-523

[28] Howe GL, Poyton HG (1960) Prevention of damage to the inferior dental nerve during the extraction of mandibular third molars. Br Dent J 109:355-363

[29] Queral-Godoy E, Valmaseda-Castellon E, Berini-Aytes L, Gay-Escoda C (2005) Incidence and evolution of inferior alveolar nerve lesions following lower third molar extraction. Oral Surg Oral Med Oral Pathol Oral Radiol Endod 99:259-264

[30] Wagner R, DeLeo JA, Coombs DW, Myers RR (1995) Gender differences in autotomy following sciatic cryoneurolysis in the rat. Physiol Behav 58:37-41

[31] Coyle DE, Sehlhorst CS, Mascari C (1995) Female rats are more susceptible to the development of neuropathic pain using the partial sciatic nerve ligation (PSNL) model. Neurosci Lett 186:135-138

[32] Heasman PA, Beynon ADG (1987) Myelinated axon counts of human inferior alveolar nerves. J Anat 151:51-56

[33] Patel SV, Mutyala S, Leske DA, Hodge DO, Holmes JM. (2004) Incidence, associations, and evaluation of sixth nerve palsy using a population-based method. Ophthalmology. 111:369-75

[34] Campbell KE, Brundage JF (2002) Effects of climate, latitude, and season on the incidence of Bell's palsy in the US armed forces, October 1997 to September 1999. Am J Epidemiol 156:32–39

[35] Monini S, Lazzarino AI, Iacolucci C, Buffoni A, Barbara M (2010) Epidemiology of Bell's palsy in an Italian Health District: incidence and case-control study. Acta Otorhinolaryngol Ital 30:198-204

[36] Tiemstra JD, Khatkhate N (2007) Bell's palsy: diagnosis and management. Am Fam Physician 76:997–1002

[37] Hullar TE, Minor LB, Zee DS (2005) Evaluation of the patient with dizziness. In: Cummings CW (ed) Cummings otolaryngology head & neck surgery, 4th edn, vol 4. Elsevier Mosby, Philadelphia, pp 3160–3198

[38] Lempert T, Neuhauser H (2009) Epidemiology of vertigo, migraine and vestibular migraine. J Neurol 256:333–338

[39] Neuhauser HK, von Brevern M, Radtke A, Lezius F, Feldmann M, Ziese T, Lempert T (2005) Epidemiology of vestibular vertigo: a neurotologic survey of the general population. Neurology 65:898-904

[40] Yin M, Ishikawa K, Wong WH, Shibata Y (2009) A clinical epidemiological study in 2169 patients with vertigo. Auris Nasus Larynx 36:30-5

[41] Wladislavosky-Waserman P, Facer GW, Mokri B, Kurland LT (1984) Menière's disease: a 30-year epidemiologic and clinical study in Rochester, Mn, 1951–1980. Laryngoscope 94:1098–1102

[42] Havia M, Kentala E, Pyykkö I (2005) Prevalence of Menie`re's disease in general population of Southern Finland. Otolaryngol Head Neck Surg 133:762–768

[43] Davis B (1987) The incidence of tinnitus. In: Slater R, Terry M (eds) Tinnitus: a guide for sufferers and professionals. Croom Helm, Beckenham, Kent, pp 88–98

[44] Graham JT (1965) Relation of tinnitus to age. Acta Otolaryngol 59(s202):24-26

[45] Coles RRA (1984) Epidemiology of tinnitus: demographic and clinical features. J Laryngol Otology (Suppl 9):195-202

[46] Møller MB, Møller AR, Jannetta PJ, Jho HD (1993) Vascular decompression surgery for severe tinnitus: Selection criteria and results. Laryngoscope 103:421–427

[47] Kacker SK (1997) Hearing impairment in the aged. Indian J Med Res 106:333-339
[48] Hinchcliffe R, Jones WI (1968) Hearing levels of a suburban Jamaican population. Int J Audiol 7:239-258
[49] Bunch CC, Raiford TS (1931) Race and sex variations in auditory acuity. Arch Otolaryngol 13:423-434
[50] Berger EH, Royster LH, Thomas WG (1977) Hearing levels of nonindustrial exposed subjects. J Occup Med 19:664-670
[51] Starr A, Picton TW, Sininger Y, Hood LJ, Berlin CI (1996) Auditory neuropathy. Brain 119:741-753
[52] Nakashima T (2001) Sudden deafness. In: Nomura Y, Komatsuzaki A, Honjyo I (eds) Clinical textbooks of the ear, nose and throat regions 21, No. 5. Nakayama Shoten Co. Ltd., Tokyo, pp 259–269 (Japanese)
[53] Araújo CG, Nobrega AC, Castro CL. (1989) Vagal activity: effect of age, sex and physical activity pattern. Braz J Med Biol Res 22:909-211
[54] Bruyn GW (1983) Glossopharyngeal neuralgia. Cephalalgia 3:143-157
[55] Kandan SR, Khan S, Jeyaretna DS, Lhatoo S, Patel NK, Coakham HB (2010) Neuralgia of the glossopharyngeal and vagal nerves: long-term outcome following surgical treatment and literature review. Br J Neurosurg 24:441-446
[56] Crue BL, Todd EM (1968) Vagal neuralgia. In: Vinken PJ, Bruyn GW (eds) Headaches and cranial neuralgias. North-Holland Pub. Co., Amsterdam, pp 362–367
[57] Rushton JG, Stevens JC, Miller RH (1981) Glossopharyngeal (vagoglossopharyngeal) neuralgia: a study of 217 cases. Arch Neurol 38:201-205
[58] Khasar SG, Isenberg WM, Miao FJ, Gear RW, Green PG, Levine JD (2001) Gender and gonadal hormone effects on vagal modulation of tonic nociception. J Pain 2:91-100
[59] Titche LL (1976) Causes of recurrent laryngeal nerve paralysis. Arch Otolaryngol 102:259-261
[60] Parnell FW, Brandenburg JH (1970) Vocal cord paralysis: A review of 100 cases. Laryngoscope 80:1036-1045.
[61] Nozoe I, Hirano M, Shin T, Maeyama T (1972) Recurrent laryngeal nerve palsy: A clinical study 400 cases. Otologia Fukuoka 18:411-417
[62] Hojyo M, Nishiyama H (1972) The statistical observation of recurrent laryngeal nerve palsy. Jpn J Natl Med Serv 26:597-601
[63] Yanohara K, Hisa Y, Suzuki Y, Mizuta Y, Matsui T, Sato F, Mizukoshi O (1978) Clinical aspect of recurrent laryngeal nerve palsy. Pract Otol Kyoto 71:1201-1207
[64] Yamada M, Hirano M, Ohkubo H (1983) Recurrent laryngeal nerve paralysis: A 10-year review of 564 patients. Auris Nasus Larynx 10(Suppl):S1-15
[65] Ishikawa T (1977) Clinical study of unilateral vocal cord paralysis: Level differences between the vocal cords. Pract Otol Kyoto 70:453-461
[66] Work WP (1941) paralysis and paresis of the vocal cords: A statistical review. Arch Otolaryngol 34:267-280
[67] Huppler EG, Schmidt HW, Devine D (1955) Causes of vocal-cord paralysis. Proc Staff Meet Mayo Clin 30:518-521